FAMILY CARE

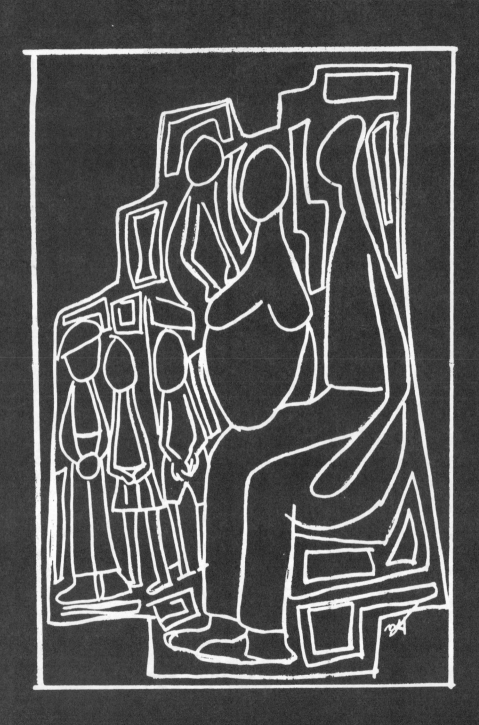

FAMILY CARE

A guide......

edited by

Naomi Baumslag, M.D.

Associate Professor of Preventive
Medicine and Community Health.
Emory University, Atlanta.

The Williams & Wilkins Company
Baltimore, Maryland.

Copyright ©, 1973
The Williams & Wilkins Company
428 E. Preston Street
Baltimore, Md. 21202, U.S.A.

Made in the United States of America

Library of Congress Catalog Card Number 73-4556
SBN 683-00412-3

Composed and printed at the
Waverly Press, Inc.
Mt. Royal and Guilford Aves.
Baltimore, Md. 21202, U.S.A.

Dedication

TO MY FAMILY, STUDENTS, COLLEAGUES AND PATIENTS, whose thoughts became written words. With Love, a word used seldom, if at all, in medical schools.

Contributors

Naomi Baumslag, M.D. Associate Professor Preventive Medicine and Community Health, Emory University, Atlanta.

John R. Boring III, Ph.D. Associate Professor Preventive Medicine and Community Health, Emory University, Atlanta.

John K. Davidson, Ph.D., M.D. Professor of Medicine and Director of Diabetes Day Care Center, Emory University, Atlanta.

Alan Drinnan, D.D.S., M.D. Professor and Chairman, Oral Medicine, School of Dentistry, State University of New York at Buffalo.

Harley Gordon, D.C.H., M.D. Chairman of Pediatrics, Catholic Medical Center of Brooklyn and Queens. Assistant Clinical Professor of Pediatrics, Downstate Medical Center, New York.

Irving Kanner, M.D. Professor of Medicine and Director of Ambulatory Care, University of Kentucky.

Zuher Naib, M.D. Professor of Pathology, Emory University, Atlanta.

Louise Rauh, M.D. Professor of Pediatrics, University of Cincinnati Medical School.

Robert M. Reece, M.D. Associate Professor of Pediatrics and Director of Community Health Services, Rockford Medical School, Illinois.

Clarice Reid, M.D. Medical Consultant to Sickle Cell Program, Department of HEW.

Kenneth B. Roberts, M.D. Chief, Physician's Development Activity, Health Professions Branch Training Program, Center for Communicable Disease Control, Atlanta.

Martin Saidleman, M.D. Assistant Professor of Pediatrics, University of Cincinnati. Associate Director of Maternal and Infant Care.

Luis Saldana, M.D. Assistant Professor of Obstetrics and Gynecology, Albert Einstein Hospital, Yeshiva University, New York.

Edward B. Silberstein, M.D. Associate Professor of Medicine and Radiology, University of Cincinnati.

Ralph E. Yodaiken, M.D. Professor of Pathology, Emory University, Atlanta.

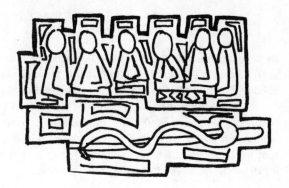

Preface

Understanding, consideration, and a knowledge of patient
values are essential ingredients in the management and treatment
of disease for the health care of communities. When the physician is called on
to make value judgements to attain consumer participation and satisfaction, these
decisions should be made in accordance with the patients' life styles. The
lower the student or physician on the totem pole, the less responsibility for such
decision making. While in a hospital setting the patient is remote; in a practice
or clinic situation he/she is dealt with directly. Hence the ability for adequate
judgement and team work is of key importance.

It is hoped that while accumulating scientific facts, the student will
develop a spirit of inquiry and will challenge dogma and ritual which does not
serve patients' medical and human needs. This book was written to encourage such
an approach by filling in the gaps left in our highly technical and fragmented
medical curricula.

The book had its origins around a core of elective seminars given to a
group of sophomore medical students. From their reports on home visits, it was clear
that terms such as "foster parent", "illegitimate", "play sister" as well as family
priorities were poorly understood. In the family clinic many students were
initially unable to make simple measurements (some had never used a tape measure,
a scale or a clinical thermometer). Nor had they been taught to comprehend
patient problems or priorities, and they were therefore unable to effectively
communicate with their patients. To many students "poverty", for example,
was a word and not a fact of life; and consequently the life style and language
of the poor was relatively incomprehensible.

With the support of some dedicated members of faculty at the Cincinnati
Medical Center, a guide for the care of families began to emerge. But it soon

became obvious that the guide should become a book that would discuss matters such as diet in relation to cultural habit; the pap smear and patient attitudes; child rearing and child abuse; biopsy techniques and the environment.

A publisher was sought who would select a different style of medical text book, written in simple language around concepts seldom discussed in the wards. Jon Davidson of Williams and Wilkins took up the challenge. It is hoped that this book will be enjoyed and added to by those who still believe that the art of medicine is as important as its science.   NB

Acknowledgements

We are grateful for students and colleagues of the Family Care
Program at the University of Cincinnati Medical School who set
the ball rolling: Raymond Suskind, Chairman of Environmental Health; Edward
Silberstein; Mrs. Eastman and Mrs. Hunter, who were staunch supporters of the
clinic in which the students worked; Marva Greene, who assisted in compilation of
the bibliography; Mervyn Susser, who generously contributed material and gave
encouragement; Joe Agranoff; George Columbel; Norman Mathews; Vickie Strobel,
Catherine Bufford and Kay Gatins, who reviewed the manuscript and added many
valuable suggestions; Roz Edell and Barbara Fothergill, who began the typing;
Susan Williams, who prepared the final camera copy and proved invaluable in many
ways; Jane Scott, who added a sense of humor and art to the existing illustrations.
Thomas F. Sellers, Chairman of the Department of Preventive Medicine and
Community Health at Emory, made the completion of this book a pleasure;
hopefully it reflects, to some extent, his interest and concern for people.

Most of all my thanks go to Ralph E. Yodaiken, my husband, whose example
encouragement, and practical advice has made this book a family venture.

The early stages of this work were supported in part by NIH Grant No. 5
DO 4 AH 00648-07 and later by Grant No. 5 DO 4 AH 00733-06.

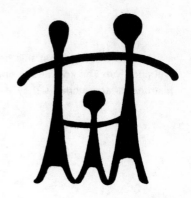

Foreword

In the early 1960's technology in medicine reigned supreme; and little attention was paid to those who knew the importance of paying attention to the patient's feelings, human behavior and the family as a unit of care. In the late 60's, for reasons not yet clear, the efforts of a few caught the public's fancy and almost overnight "comprehensive care" and "family medicine" became a major force in medical education.

Academic institutions were caught unprepared for the sudden change of course. Medical colleges were being called upon to teach a discipline, family medicine, for which there existed little scientific information. This was made all the more difficult by the lack of faculty members interested in or knowledgeable about primary health care. In short, there was no research background, existing scientific literature or body of knowledge upon which to base a course in family medicine.

Those teachers brave enough to engage themselves with students found they were called upon to teach what they did not know and to serve as a role model for a physician that did not exist. The authors of this handbook on family care are such teachers, and have had to draw on their personal experience and intuition in preparing it. In particular, the handbook represents the distillation of the experiences of a warm, gifted and observant physician, Dr. Naomi Baumslag. While it might be easy to question some of the statements made, to do so is to forget that in primary care it is the process, not the content, that helps the patient. It is not so important what is done as it is how it's done.

xiii

It is my hope that this handbook will grow and that the students who use it will add to it. The knowledge and skills they acquire will soon exceed that of their instructors, and, perhaps they will produce a textbook of family medicine.

Lynn R. Carmichael, M.D.
Professor & Chairman
Dept. of Family Medicine
University of Miami

Contents

CONTENTS

CHAPTER 1

The Family

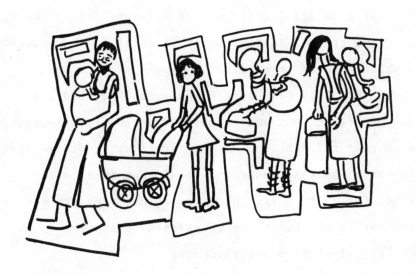

THE ELEMENTARY OR nuclear family (mother, father, child) is universal![8] Its stability and the degree of organization may vary. The family is biological[14] as no other grouping, industrial, occupational or social can claim to be; its ill-defined and amorphous structure with grand-parents, parents, children and collateral links through marriage, is a phenomenon of growth: bound together by a mixture of economic and emotional services and pooled resources - with its own mores and government.[14]

1

Families throughout the world exhibit a variety of internal kinship systems, values, beliefs and therefore motivation.[7,12] They may be small and circumscribed as in the western world or, as in the East, extended to include many relatives and even strangers. In the USA many Black families still have extended families.   The extended family may live in one home or in a family compound, or it may be distributed throughout a rural community.

Relationships between men and women, attitudes to children, and the respect and support given to grandparents depend on cultural modes. In some societies, children work early while in others education continues after maturity. In some, the cult of lifelong marriage is very strong; in others marriage rituals are breaking down as new and more compelling ideologies are taken up.

Communal type living as seen in Israel and China allows children to be cared for at an early age by other parties. Parental dependency on the other hand is much more marked in western societies where isolated nuclear families exist. In polygamous African societies a man has many wives and each wife lives in her own housing unit with her children. All the units are close together within the same compound. In this type of society men do "men's work" such as hunting and building, and women do the cooking, planting, and child-rearing. In China job discrimination on the basis of sex is virtually a thing of the past. In polygamous African society, women are married off in exchange for cattle and children are valued as providers of aged parents. In western society insurance policies or retirement funds are subscribed to in order to perpetuate a state of independence as long as possible.

It is not surprising that attitudes to sex, work, eating, child rearing, sleeping patterns, care of the aged and ill, and availability and selection of medical care are all influenced by the structure of the family.

SYNCRETIZATION

The culture of our society although uncompromising and enduring is constantly undergoing change, taking in and absorbing new ideas when these do not conflict with fundamental tenets - a process described as syncretization.[4] All new ideas are first valued according to existing ones; those which have an affinity with something in the existing culture will be most readily accepted.

THE FAMILY HISTORY

As has been pointed out a family may be nuclear and relatively small or extended and large. In the latter, an individual may be called aunt or uncle or granny and yet not be related in the true sense. (This is common in many African tribes.) To attach any significance to a positive family history requires screening of relatives and definition of

what constitutes a positive family history. The family history is always asked for in chronic diseases such as diabetes
coronary artery disease, and hypertension. Different patterns of inheritance have been ascribed to these diseases
but it may be that environmental factors are as important as
genetic factors. Therefore, in planning a family history,
the family should be clearly defined and at best include
only grandparents, parents, and offspring.[2] The larger the
number of relatives, and as in diabetes, the older the group
studied, the more chance of finding "a positive family history". Sometimes endless digging for information about
diseases with obscure genetic transmission may cause unnecessary concern in a family unless the dubious mode of inheritance is made clear to the family at the time.

FAMILY ORGANIZATION

When a man and woman have children they assume new ti-
tles, "mother" and "father". They also have additional responsibilities and added roles. In evaluating a family it is
helpful to determine whether there is deprivation, deficiency,
and dependency (family symptoms). A child may be considered
deprived if one or both parents are not present in the home.
Deficiency exists if there is inadequate shelter, food or
clothing. If a family is not able to provide for itself and
has to obtain assistance from the community for health care
and living allowance, then this constitutes dependency.

Court[5] found a strong positive correlation between family symptoms and the higher incidence of growth failure, severe lower respiratory tract infections, gastroenteritis, squint, and enuresis. Parents are often not able to cope with their problems and at the same time remain loyal to their responsibilities. For good child care, parents need to 1) be present 2) provide adequate material care 3) participate in family life and 4) establish satisfactory personal relationships. The neighborhood school, town and nation all have their impact on the family.

CHILD REARING

To assess child care practices the physician needs to know child development, cultural mores and family dynamics. The family perpetuates its attitudes through child rearing. In the nuclear family the load of responsibility is greater than that of the extended family. This is even more so in single parent homes (unwed mothers, divorced or separated). It has always been assumed that the natural parents are the best caretakers. However more evidence is accumulating to show that this is not always so and the rising incidence of child abuse may be a direct correlation. Dawson[6] documented that the state of motherhood has undergone change. A mother has never been so alone as in western society. Modern life has placed intolerable burdens on the mother of a young family - burdens she often carries alone. As a single parent she may have endless financial problems. Even though she may come from a large family, relatives may live far away or be too busy to help her. Since one in four marriages end in divorce and our attitudes to "illegitimacy" are changing, there are an increasing number of single parents found. With the newer social structure, the family is becoming smaller and absence of the male in the household more frequent.

The "extended" or three-generation family often presents difficulties in Western society. The grandmother, who may shoulder the main responsibility for child rearing, cannot legally act as decision maker in the case of medical emergencies.

There are certain situations where child rearing stress may be accentuated. Look for them in a mother who has or has had:

1. frequent pregnancies (several pre-school children at home)

2. premature, physically or mentally handicapped child

3. a child out of wedlock

4. an absent husband   a) <u>physically</u> - due to demands of job, service;   b) <u>psychologically</u> - because of the "television sitter"

5. financial strain

6. emotionally or mentally retarded parents

7. a history of alcohol or drug abuse

8. marital discord

Parental neglect may be suspected if evidence of uncleanliness below the level of the parent's cultural and economic standards is observed. Uncut dirty nails, dirty clothes, no shoes, neglected cradle cap, impetigo or ammonial diapers should all raise questions about the quality of home care. Failure to thrive, once organic causes are excluded, should also alert the physician. Emotional deprivation may also be evident.

FAMILY ADJUSTMENTS TO GROWTH AND CHANGE

Olsen[13] has drawn attention to several characteristics among families making positive adjustments to daily stress. In these families there is a clear separation of the generations so that the parents are satisfying each other's emotional need. In the case of conflict, they are able to fight straight and don't involve the children as allies. There is also a flexibility within the family and between roles so that shifting can be tolerated with relative comfort. There is a tolerance for individuation. The family can accept and enjoy differences in the behavior and attitudes to the individual members. Communications among the family members are direct and consistent and tend to confirm the self esteem of each.

FAMILY CRISIS

At certain times the family may have to deal with additional stress which may be short term (an acute illness,

a birth, a divorce, a death) or long term (an adjustment to
chronic illness, loss of limb, a mental or other physical
handicap). When such a crisis is being dealt with satisfactorily the following healthy pattern is evident:[9]

1. An initial period of stunned denial. The family
    can't hear what is being said to them.

2. A period of confusion, anxiety and frequently re-
    sentment of the sick family member.

3. A period of recovery and reorganization.

Supporting help which you might supply depends on the
stage of stress. Professional support can alleviate a lot
of unnecessary strain and facilitate readjustment. In the
case of the chronically ill, people with increased dependence
a considerable burden is placed on the family.[1] Bear in mind
that the sickness of one individual is the family's illness
as well. In some cases a relative may need as much care as
the patient and this should not be forgotten either.[3,15]   At
these times the physician may be the emotional anchor on
which the family depends.[15]

However, watching a patient with a progressive disease
deteriorate on a therapeutic regime is not easy and physician
as well as nursing personnel may become anxious, depressed an
irritable.[11]   There is a need to discuss their own feelings
with each other in order to deal positively with the family.
Ignoring this problem will not solve it; but frank open discussion may help significantly.

REFERENCES

1. Baumslag N, Yodaiken RE: Care of special people. New
    Eng J Med 286:1220, 1972 (Letter)

2. Baumslag N, Yodaiken RE, Varady J: Standardization of
    terminology in diabetes: Types and family history.
    Diabetes 119:664, 1970

3. Binger CM, Ablin AR, Fewerstein RC, Kushner JH: Child-
    hood leukemia: Emotional impact on patient and family.
    New Eng J Med 280:414, 1969

4. Brockington F: Family life. World Health. London,
    Churchill, 1967

5. Court SDM: Child health in a changing community. Brit
    Med J 2:125, 1971

6. Dawson D: The Scotsman. Jan 19, 1970

7. Elliot K: The Family and Its Future CIBA Foundation
    Symposium. London, Churchill, 1970

8. Firth R: The child and its relationship to the commu-
    nity. International Child Welfare Review 9:123-136,
    1953

9. Hill R: Social stresses on the family. Social Case
    Work 39:139, 1958

10. Andreasen NJC, et al: Management of emotional reactions
    in seriously burned adults. New Eng J Med 286:65, 1972

11. Martin HL, Lawrie JH, Wilkinson AW: The family of the
    fatally burned child. Lancet 2:628, 1968

12. Mead M, Heyman K: The Family. New York, MacMillan
    Company, 1965

13. Olsen EH: The impact of serious illness on the family.
    Postgrad Med 47:169, 1970

14. Susser MW, Watson W: The Cycle of Family Development
    in Sociology in Medicine. Second edition. London,
    Oxford University Press, 1971

15. Zachary RB: Ethical and social aspects of the treatment
    of spina bifida. Lancet 2:274, 1968.

CHAPTER 2

Home and the Community

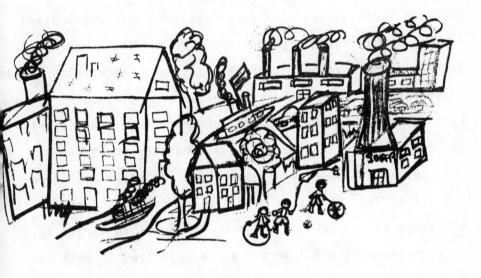

FOR EFFECTIVE PREVENTION and therapy the individual
should be seen in his or her milieu. Only then
can the impact of the numerous environmental factors be
evaluated and this knowledge used to implement total care
for the family. Even a detailed social or family history
does not replace a home visit. In fact, much more effort is
needed to interview patients on their home ground than in a
captive situation such as outpatient clinic or in a hospital
setting. It is important to appreciate that isolated facts

obtained from the hospital patient may cover the major medical problems but will not reveal the total patient-picture.

ATTITUDES

Subconsciously people attempt to impose their own socio-economic system, cultural values and attitudes on those with different life styles. In many cases one has preconceived notions of how certain groups function and these may be theoretical and vague rather than factual. Because the needs of people vary, it is always necessary for the doctor to become fully acquainted with the community he is dealing with and to determine the cultural components of the group.

Sexual attitudes are related to life style and education; therefore to expect middle class morality from families who sleep in one room is unreal. Attitudes to virginity, rape, pregnancy, and love are all deeply tied in with the culture. Rather than searching out the weaknesses, look for family strength and lack of obsessive compulsiveness.

The problem that continually crops up is a definition of poverty.[7] The interpretation of poverty depends on education and experience. For instance, in a word association test using the word "poverty", we found that the poor used descriptive associations such as "no money", "no home", "no clothes", "no food", while psychiatric residents (even more than medical students) used intellectualizations such as "disenfranchised", "ghetto", "welfare", "deprivation",

POVERTY-(ANALYSIS OF FREE ASSOCIATION)

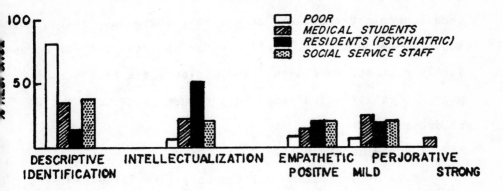

BAUMSLAG & WINGET

"socio-economic", and even "Biafra". Perjoratives such as "unsanitary", "filth", "lack of motivation" were also used. In delivery of health care an assessment must be made of the patient's own concepts, priorities and attitudes.

To some students, residents and teachers, poverty is associated with a set of circumstances that implies only the dark, wet, starving or thin. Poverty [12] in the presence of material assets is incomprehensible. But welfare patients or people with low incomes egged on by high-pressure sales-men tend to buy television sets or cars on credit with high interest rates and subsequently find themselves harassed by bill collectors. To such poor people, a Cadillac or a "prin-cess" telephone gives the status they have no other way of achieving even if this social elevation is temporary and

soon lost because of forfeiture clauses in the contract.
For a brief time they may enjoy the envy of others in the
same economic bracket who do not have these luxuries. Clothe
too, may be deceptive. Well dressed patients are not necessarily rich any more than "hip" patients are necessarily
poor. Life style and economic pressures dictate the type
of dress.

FAMILY PLANNING AND HEALTH

It is often stated that the poor like large families,
and that family planning will deprive them of an area of
creativity. It may be that among the poor the stigma of
infertility is higher and that the religious edicts and fear
of the unknown is greater. There is also a fear of genocide.
The Black male may be afraid that birth control is an attempt
to reduce the number of Blacks. It is always preferable to
probe attitudes before pushing cures. Certain questions
need to be asked - what is the attitude to the present pregnancy and to further pregnancies? Are more children wanted
and if not, what birth control measures are being considered?
Has anyone in the family had venereal disease? Are there
any special or unconventional preventive measures being used?

The use of health facilities is also pertinent to the
well-being of the present or future family. The number of
children who have received all their immunizations is an
index of utilization of preventive medical care. Adults who

use emergency services all the time are less likely to devote time to check-up visits. Handicapped members of the family - C. P. (cerebral palsy), deaf, blind, mentally retarded, congenital heart patients, those who have had disabling trauma or elective amputations - also have a significant effect on the health attitudes of the family and this may depend on the way in which the disabled member was handled by a hospital or specific agency.

Many families doctor themselves or seek advice from the local pharmacist. Exotic advertisements or lenient doctors may lead to the habitual use of tranquilizers, or "pain killers" to control "nerves". At all socio-economic levels, people are frequently unaware of the need to adopt preventive care measures. They may be too busy, too concerned with health fads or spurious "medical advisors", or they may be "hooked" on alcohol patent medicines or drugs and unable or afraid to use available medical facilities.

Economics and Reasons for Visiting the Doctor

Although it is repeatedly stated that health care is a right and not a privilege, in practice many people cannot afford this "right". The source of a patient's finance may be as a wage-earner or as a recipient of financial aid from Welfare, Aid to Dependent Children (ADC), Aid for the Blind or some other program. The fact that a person is receiving aid does not mean it is adequate because it takes an

experienced, astute person to budget adequately and compe-
tently. Money can be saved by buying milk powder instead of
milk, and yet not everyone likes the taste of milk powder or
the bother involved in its preparation. The source of income sometimes determines which forms of health care are
available. Indigent patients are often treated only in specified hospitals. Financial or religious restrictions may
bar these patients from other hospitals.

People come to doctors with an endless variety of problems but the driving force is sometimes well concealed. One
mother may bring her child or come herself to the doctor for
the slightest ailment - afraid of diabetes or tuberculosis
which had previously appeared in a relative. Another patient
will only come to a hospital when the pain or discomfort is
too severe to bear any longer. Frequently the latter patient is afraid of modern medical practices or hospital costs
and may have been in the hands of the local herb-man, medicine man, "medical advisor", or whatever, for some time.

When a group of mothers attending a family clinic with
their newborns were asked what problems most commonly brought
patients to the hospital, they gave the following replies
most frequently: the pill, missed period, pregnancy, bleedin
unbearable pain. A group of medical students (attending the
same clinic) answering the same question listed the following: "they need wiser medical advise"; "need for

counseling"; "health certificates"; "they are hypochondriacs".
Both groups agreed that immunizations and trauma were common
reasons for attendance. At that particular clinic it cost
$10.00 per person per visit. The $10.00 priorities of the
students did not match the $10.00 priorities of the patients.
Where there is no family fee, preventive health care can be
too expensive for people with more pressing priorities.

LIFE STYLES

The life style of the "family" in the home, apartment,
or multiple dwelling has a bearing on the family's health.
The priority of care, the level of education, the income and
the social way of life are all important to delivery and
utilization of health care. Race and religion, and most of
all, economic bracket contribute to a life style which may
manifest itself in speech, dress, diet, drinking, smoking
and child rearing practices.

In some societies illness is believed to be punishment
for wrongs and is associated with guilt. The local herb man
may be used to treat many conditions; also home remedies are
passed on from one generation to another. Among the Navaho
Indians illness is usually ascribed to the breaking of one
of the taboos which guide the behavior of the Navaho.[1] Illness, therefore, may be due to contact with the ghosts of
the dead, or even the bad wishes of another Navaho who has
resorted to witchery. In this Indian culture religion and

medicine are inseparable. Mexican families often have a
sister who is the tia (aunt). This member of the family
helps out during illness, delivery or any significant family
event. She is rewarded with gifts. In one case where food
was usually the gift, the tia became obese. Being aware of
this custom, the physicians asked the relatives to reward
the tia in another way so she could reduce her weight and
possibly improve her hypertension. The Eskimo treats ear-
ache with warm seal oil and joint pain with willow bark in-
fusions. The willow bark contains salicylic acid.

Such customs are not limited to specific tribes or
religious groups or to underdeveloped or economically deprived people. Similar practices are common in rural America
It may be an error to assume that your immaculate city patient is sticking to her salt-free diet. If you ask her to
empty her purse, perhaps you'd be surprised to find tins or
bags of baking powder which she takes in large quantities
for all her aches and pains.

DIET AND NUTRITION

Diet is discussed in detail elsewhere but a few points
are pertinent here. Eating habits must be taught in terms
of a culture. The people of Yucatan took pride in the produc
tion of white tortillas which were made by mixing corn meal
with lime, boiling it, and letting the mixture soak overnight. Although the whitened meal was a source of satisfacti

to the family, it was a matter of concern as the process de-
stroyed niacin in the meal and this deficiency caused pel-
lagra. The Mayans were told that they would require pills
of niacinamide or injections if they persisted in bleaching
the corn meal. Despite the warning, it was found later that
the people had reverted to soaking the meal with lime because
some millers had complained that the unwhitened meal clogged
their grinding equipment. So the education had to be re-
sumed. This illustrates the necessity of understanding and
working closely with the culture to achieve desired results.[11]

It is impractical to tell a Hindu patient that meat is
a good source of protein or a northerner that hog maw (stomach) is cheap and also a good protein source as southerners
well know. Don't advise a pensioner to eat a balanced diet
unless you know he has the money to buy a balanced diet. To
get an idea of the typical daily or weekly diet, ask the
mother for a rough outline of a week's menu and the approximate quantity of milk, meat and eggs purchased. Inquire as
to dietary cravings during pregnancy. Sometimes during pregnancy patients develop a distinct distaste for foods. They
may not eat salads or meat and no amount of persuasion will
make them add substances not normally eaten to their daily
intake. The pregnant female may exhibit cravings. Pica,
the habitual, purposeful, and compulsive search for and ingestion of such non-food items as laundry starch, magnesium

carbonate, earth and kleenex tissues, may develop. When
this takes the form of ice eating, it is called pagophagia.[1]
Some investigators believe it is related to iron deficiency
and that treatment with iron stops the craving for these
substances. In addition to harming the mother, the ingestion of toxic substances may harm the fetus.

Pica eating in children is associated with paint, plaster and batteries - all good sources of lead poisoning.[9] In
poorly nourished children it is not unusual to see evidence
of vitamin deficiencies, malnutrition and dental caries.
Apathy and poor learning are consequences of bad diet as
well as the lack of loving care!

Knowing about the usual diet, its deficiencies, excesses
and quirks, allows the physician to prescribe palatable and
economically feasible substitutes and additives such as iron,
Vitamin B_{12} and folic acid.

HOUSING

Valuable clues can be obtained by finding out if a home
is urban or rural and the location in relation to traffic
and factories. The street address sometimes indicates the
economic bracket but the size of the house may be deceptive.
The number of mailboxes may give a clue as to the number of
families living in a house even if they are not all seen
during the visit. The appearance of the residence and a
garden may also be helpful. The presence of a zinc bathtub

hanging on a hook may suggest that no bathroom is present. The approximation to stores or industry should be noted. A railway line or factory may produce air pollutants, and consequently, be related to allergy or chronic lung disease. Homeowners usually take better care of their own property. On a visit, take special notice of peeling paint which often contains lead or patchy plaster. In some rural areas, out- side fireplaces are a "burn" hazard. As a word of warning, remember that a clean and neat exterior with potted plants may be as deceptive of the inside conditions as a ramshackle exterior with old cars and broken bottles.

Where septic tanks are used and there is seepage of sewage into water supplies, outbreaks of diseases such as infectious hepatitis can occur. This is particularly preva- lent during the rainy season and it is pollution of this type that occurs among rich and poor.

The type of housing is important. Children in apart- ments with no outdoor play area and no balcony become iso- lated, especially in cold climates, and for them the "world" is small and restricted and personal experience and relation- ships with others are limited.[10] On the other hand, wooded areas carry problems such as poison ivy and Rocky Mountain spotted fever.

Poor hygienic facilities encourage rats, and mites and skin infestation such as scabies (caused by a mite Sarcoptes

scabei) may be seen. Pediculosis (lice) are frequently en-
countered among people whose clothing is infrequently washed
and changed and with whom bathing is not a regular habit -
especially elderly people!

The inside of a house and its contents also contribute
to the assessment of family values. Books, record albums,
pictures, models, plants and pets indicate a way of life.
Many children grow up with fake plants or even fake fish.
This affects tactile, sensory and auditory perception and
color attitudes. Poor lighting too may affect vision. Constantly watching television results in "people deprivation"
and real-life discussions, conversations and games are
limited. The children grow up with make believe values and
false impressions of what constitutes "good" or "bad". Thei
social conduct, reactions to pain and treatment, may all be
conditioned by their television education.

Maps, charts and photographs are useful adjuncts when
making a meaningful record. Permission slips must be signed
before any photographs are taken of the patients.

HOUSEHOLD

In considering the family, therefore, note where they
live and for how long they have occupied the house; what
kind of living facilities are available and how they are
utilized; the number of householders and their permanence
(loose male-female relationships may result in frequent

changes of address); the type of family associations such as
in a single or multiple family. Do the parents or grandparents live with the family in the same house (communal
living), or in close proximity to relatives (isolated or
group living)? The reasons for family inter-relationships
are pertinent, too. People may live in groups for economic
reasons. It may be as well to consider why the rich live
as isolated elementary family units.

Adopted children in the household may be badly treated
or emotionally deprived. Since many associations are out of
wedlock, it is not rare to find a "battered" adopted child
in a loose-linked arrangement. Furthermore, a genetic history from a family where all the children are of different
paternal origin will give spurious inheritance patterns.
This is particularly true if the mother deliberately or un-
wittingly conceals the fact that the children had different
fathers. It may take considerable time and patience to con-
struct an accurate genetic tree.

SOME FACTS AND FIGURES

At present, for the poor, the risk of dying under the
age of 25 is four times the national average. Life expectancy among the non-white population is 63.6 years as compared to 70.2 years in whites. Maternal mortality among
non-whites is 90.2 per 100,000 as compared to 22.4 per
100,000 in whites. The infant mortality rate of non-whites

is greater than in whites. According to the United States
Children's Bureau, infant mortality rises as family income
decreases. Fifty per cent of poor children are incompletely
immunized against smallpox or measles. Sixty per cent of
poor children have never seen a dentist. Operative procedures, such as appendectomy and tonsillectomy, are commoner
among the middle class than among the poor.[2]

THE INTERVIEW

The most important part of interviewing is listening.[3,6]
Do not interrogate the patient but carefully follow a line
of questioning. This is an art developed by conscious experience and needs a lot of practice. No one person has the
same approach. Sometimes the interviewer has to change his
tactics according to the type of person being interviewed;
this is called the "chameleon" approach.

Remember that no one remembers lots of detail unless it
is of prime importance to the person. Milestones may be
important to one mother and not to another depending on
factors such as education, number of children and the amount
of leisure. The ability to observe is related to leisure
time which, in turn, may be dependent on economic conditions.

Terminology depends on education, culture and age
group. "Falling out" may mean lightheaded, vertigo, syncope
or epilepsy; "a shot" is an injection; "stoned" used to mean
drunk - now it means drugged; "haircut" means syphilis; the

"clap", "drop" or "running rains" - gonorrhea; "whites" is
leukorrhea; "hives" - allergy; "cascade" - vomit; "crabs" -
lice; loss of "nature" - impotence. To an American a "rubber" is a condom - to an Englishman, it means eraser. An
Englishwoman talks of a "napkin" which in America is a diaper. An Appalachian talks of pain that "sprangles" which
means spreads, and "misery", to some, means pain. The patient and doctor often communicate at different levels.[4]
Constipation may mean decreased, difficult bowel action to
the surgeon. To the patient it may mean hard stools, or the
inability to have a bowel motion daily. Substituting "loose
stools" for diarrhea or "tiredness" for fatigue can make for
comprehension and better communication.

An interview can be regarded as a piece of sculpture.
The appreciation of what is said or observed will vary from
one individual to another.[5] Not all will see the same angles
and shadows, curves and patterns. A more enterprising and
inquiring approach may reveal more than obvious facts or
repeated exposure in the same settings may bring out facets·
of life which are at first concealed in the shadows, such as
marital friction, abnormal behavior patterns or the advantages and disadvantages of a particular home environment.

POINTERS IN A HOME VISIT

If both parents are available, try and make an appointment at a time that both can be met. A street address can

be misleading so don't arrive expecting a destitute family
or be upset if you find material assets where you least
expect them. Be "human" and start with a friendly greeting.
Notice the clothing and appearance of the mother and decide
if she's apprehensive, friendly or sullen.

You have not come to impose your way of living or your
standards; nor are you there to pass judgment on morals or
political views or to alter living conditions without being
asked. If a young mother has five illegitimate children
and doesn't use birth control measures, you could tell her
what measures are available but should not tell her that she
must use one of the methods. Marriage is a required social
custom in some groups but in others illegitimacy is equally
acceptable and does not carry a social stigma.

Financial facts can be obtained with help of the social
worker or from the hospital chart. The people seen at
"charity" hospitals have been repeatedly evaluated as to
their financial status and expenditures. Welfare patients
are checked before delivery for prenatal or postnatal care
charges and if a card is mislaid or lost, they are usually
reevaluated.

Be completely unbiased in reporting the home visit.[8]
Don't present "loaded" data without a thought to the interpretation. For example:

Family	Mother's age and marital status	Dependency	Mother's Education
A	Unmarried 40 years	On welfare 3 or 4 <u>children</u> (Husband?)	(Drop out)
B	Married 40 years	4 young children supported by husband and self. Husband is a teacher.	Librarian

If information of this type is given to a visiting
nurse or social worker, it can be misleading and produce unfortunate results for the family. Family "A" may be considered as socially unacceptable by an "uptight" prospective
interviewer and will not stand a chance of receiving sympathetic assistance. Family "B" may be considered "respec-
table" and "worthy" of assistance. Consequently, both
families may be handled differently. These examples illus-
trate how biased information can influence attitudes.

A patient has the right to choose a doctor but sometimes this right cannot be realized for financial reasons.
If the doctor or student cannot communicate; or feels a lack
of trust or mutual respect; or if either becomes angry with
the other, it is better to recommend that the patient see
someone else. Not everyone would agree with this point of
view. But there are few clear cut rules in medicine and the

home visit should be friendly and nonjudgmental of the patient's life style. The real questions is - can this family
be helped in any way? Not - does this family match my concept of a worthy cause?

SUMMARY

A "good history" given in compliance with the demand of
a doctor in a hospital or clinic and in a time of stress may,
in fact, lead to false impressions. A history does not replace a home visit for both are essential and augment each
other. A good home visit can save a lot of unnecessary
questions if the observer is astute and achieves mutual trust
and confidence. Over a succeeding number of visits a definite family pattern may emerge.

In our search for improved health care delivery, a new
style of doctor is needed - one who can work effectively as
a member of a medical team. New systems will develop as
students are exposed to the stimuli and pressures outside a
hospital setting.

FAMILY STUDY GUIDE

This set of GUIDELINES can be used to help ascertain some of the factors in health delivery and utilization. A lot of answers can be obtained without direct questioning but by observation alone. The list can be considered as a "thought-list".

Date:
Name of Family:

Address (present, past):

      How long have you lived here?
      How many times have you moved in the last 3 years?

Telephone number:

Home: Owned/rented   Monthly payment:

Transportation: own auto/neighbor's auto/bus line/taxi

Home Environment and Community

      rural/urban/factories
      Housing: public/private
              single dwelling/apartment (levels/stairs)
      Does the area provide personal safety?
      Distance:
            school/shops/clinic/physician's office/hospital

Neighborhood:

      pleasant/unpleasant/paved roads/pollution/noise
      odors
      open fire.............outhouse...............
      traffic patterns
      pets..................

Outside appearance of home:

      neat/untidy/peeling paint/broken windows/broken cars
      Water: city supply/piped inside house/well

Inside appearance of home:

      clean/dirty/untidy/sparse/crowded/dry/stuffy/other....
      Number of rooms:
      Number of occupants:

Bathrooms:
Distance of bedrooms to toilet:
Adequacy of:
      (1) heating - gas/water/electric/stove
      (2) living space
      (3) food for family
      (4) clothing
      (5) washing facilities
      (6) lighting

Reading? no/yes Type: paper/comics/books/magazines

Where are poisons and medicines kept?

Attitude towards home: ashamed/proud/apologetic/other

Relationship to neighbors:
      hostile/indifferent/friendly/close as family

Members of Household:

Relationship to Household Head	Age	Sex	Marital Status S/M/D/W*	Educ	Occupation	Remarks +H

*S=single M=married D=divorced W=widow
+H=handicapped; X=head of household

Family Tree (Example):

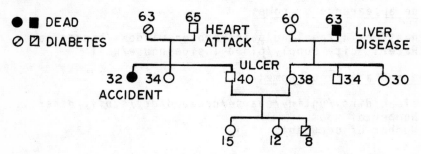

COMMUNITY RESOURCES:

Medical

Where does the family get health care?
( ) private physician ( ) health department ( ) hospital
(city, community) ( ) health center ( ) voluntary health
agency ( ) other

Immunizations of children and dates. Are they complete?
no/yes   If not, state reasons.

Name of Child	Age	DPT *	OPV *	T	Measles	Rubella	Mumps

*Indicate boosters if given
T=Tuberculin

Dental Care: provided by ( ) clinic ( ) private dentist
fillings/extractions/dentures/gum problems

Health of Family:

Genetic or familial diseases
Past illnesses (major/minor):
Operations/Accidents/Injuries:
Present illnesses (therapy?)
Bleeding tendency, healing of wounds?

Nutritional Adequacy:

Utilization of food stamp program? no/yes
Type of foods around (luxury items?)
Source of groceries and supplies:
Is diet adequate?

Non-Medical

Religious & Recreational:

Churchgoer: no/yes   Denomination:

What recreational facilities are used?

Habits: cigarettes/pipe/alcohol/drugs/over the counter
          purchases/other..........

FINANCIAL:

Source of family income: wage/social security/welfare/
                           none/other..........

Wage earners	Occupation	Work*			
Mother		P	T	pt	ft
Father		P	T	pt	ft
Other		P	T	pt	ft

                                    *P=Permanent
                                     T=Temporary
                                     pt=part-time
                                     ft=full-time

Health care paid by:

CHILD CARE:

    Major care of child by: parent/s   foster care
                              relative (specify)
    Attitude towards children:
    Protective/demanding/permissive/abusive/affectionate/
    other...................

    Who babysits?
    Children left alone: never/rarely/often

Assessment:

    1.   Deprivation (absence of a parent or both parents)

    2.   Deficiency
         A.   Shelter, food or clothing

         B.   Parent/child relationship
              Atitude to new baby or sick child

    3.   Dependency of family on community resources or
         agencies

Check:

1.   Progress of patient

2.   Family's reaction to the new baby or patient's
      return from hospital

During stress is the family

1.   At the stage of active denial of the problem.....

2.   Showing resentment and aggression towards the ill
      member of the family......

3.   Reorganizing and functioning......

Suggestions for further management (Where will follow-up
care be provided?)

How do you propose working with them?

Would a team effort help? no/yes

State if you would involve: a social worker/public health
nurse/a therapist (physio/speech)/ or anyone else to improve
the care

Which agency could provide additional care?

Suggestions for Health Education:

1.   Baby well care
2.   Accident prevention
3.   Immunizations
4.   Family planning
5.   Nutrition
6.   Other.............

REFERENCES

1. Adair J, Deuschle K, McDermott W: Patterns of health
    and disease among the Navahos. Ann Amer Acad Polit
    Soc Sci 311:86, 1957

2. Bergner L, Yerby AS: Low income and barriers to use of
    health services. New Eng J Med 278:541, 1968

3. Blum LH: Reading between the Lines. New York, Inter-
    national University Press, 1972

4. Boyl CM: Differences between patients and doctors
    interpretation of some common medical terms. Brit Med
    J 2:247, 1970

5. Francis V, Korsch BM, Morris MJ: Gaps in the doctor
    patient communication. New Eng J Med 280:535, 1969

6. Garret A: Interviewing: Its Principles and Methods.
    Family Service Association of America, 1942

7. Irelan LM: Low Income Life Styles. Publication 14,
    Division of Research, 1966

8. Knutson AL: The Individual, Society and Health Behavior
    New York, Russell Sage Foundation, 1965

9. Lanzkowsky: Investigation into the aetiology and treat-
    ment of pica. Archives of Diseases in Childhood 34:
    140, 1959

10. Life in flats. Brit Med J 1:661, 1970 (Editorial)

11. Malnutrition as a matter of taste knows no borders.
    Medical News. JAMA 216:2080, 1971

12. McMahon A, Shore MF: Some psychological reactions to
    working with the poor. Arch Gen Psychiat 18:563, 1968

13. Reynolds RD, et al: Pagophagia and iron deficiency
    anemia. Ann Int Med 69:435, 1968

SUGGESTED READING

1. Balint M: The Doctor, His Patient, and the Illness.
    New York, Internat Univ Press, 1972

2. Blum R: The Management of the Doctor-Patient Relation-
    ship. New York, McGraw-Hill, 1960

3. Cartwright A: Patients and Their Doctors: A Study of
    General Practice. London, Routledge, 1967

4. Clark M: Health in the Mexican American Culture.
    Berkeley, University of California Press, 1959

5. Freidson E: Patient's View of Medical Practice. New
    York, Russell Sage Foundation, 1961

6. Jaco EG: Patients, Physicians and Illness. New York,
    Free Press, 1958

7. Koos E: The Health in Regionsville: What the People
    Thought and Did about It. New York, Columbia University
    Press, 1954

8. Leo PA, Rosen G: A bookshelf on poverty and health.
    AJPH 59:591, 1969

9. Mechanic D: Medical Sociology: A Selective View. New
    York, Free Press, 1968

10. Medicine in the Ghetto. Edited by JC Norman. New York,
    Appleton, Century, Crofts, 1969

11. Poverty and Health: A Sociological Analysis. Edited
    by J Kosa, A Antonovsky, I Zola. Cambridge, Harvard
    University Press, 1969

12. Rogers CR: Characteristics of a helping relationship.
    Personnel and Guidance Journal 37:6, 1958

13. Saunders L: Cultural Difference and Medical Care: The
    Case of Spanish Speaking People in the Southwest. New
    York, Russell Sage Foundation, 1954

Some Thoughts on Attitudes and Cultures

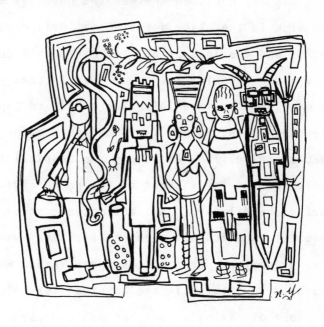

IN WESTERN CULTURE painless labor is "the thing". Whereas, previously only "obstetrical problem deliveries" were clear-cut indications for obstetrical intervention or pain killers, nowadays in many institutions obstetricians will not deliver an infant without resorting to procedures such as spinal anaesthesia or some other form of anaesthesia. The more sophisticated the

37

society, it appears, the greater number of procedures performed. Natural childbirth[3] or husband-coached natural
childbirth[1] is not encouraged in many hospitals. Unfortunately, some of the drugs and pain killers used as adjuncts
to the delivery may have harmful effects on the fetus.

One may question whether the hospital which deals with
the sick is the place for a normal delivery. The bright
lights and the lack of privacy makes this unnatural or "super
natural". "Rooming in" is allowed in some institutions but
in most, mothers and infants are handled separately, irre-
spective of the mother's wishes. One mother who had husband-
coached childbirth had to pay the hospital fifty dollars
extra for the "privilege" of having her husband with her
during the delivery. Her estimated cost of delivery in the
hospital in which not even an episiotomy was performed, was
seventy dollars per pound, and her infant weighed eleven
pounds! She stayed in the hospital for only three days.
The cost of having a baby has mounted astronomically, and
yet in frontier days, one could have a baby by natural childbirth for no cost at all. At that time, however, one out of
fifteen mothers died in childbirth. Maybe mothers needing
help should be evaluated more critically and separated from
those who can deliver with a minimum amount of interference.

Natural delivery is achieved in a number of ways. In
our system the woman lies on her back and pushes from a

reclining position. In most primitive societies, the women
squat. In our society, delivery is a hospital event. But
it was not always so. In earlier days as in many other cultures nowadays, the women of the family or tribe assist with
the delivery. In some African societies "Nyangas" or "San-
gomas", self-trained midwives are called in to assist with
the delivery. Sometimes if they are impatient they urge
the women to bear down prematurely and thus produce serious
complications such as - cervical edema, lacerations and even
uterine rupture. In our society we use Oxytocin (Pitocin)
drips to hasten labor. We are aware of one hospital where
patients close to term were given Pitocin on Thursday morning
to insure that the obstetrician was not disturbed over the
weekend!

Infant mortality is high among African tribes for a
variety of reasons - poor nutrition sepsis both in mother
and child and uneducated delivery.[9] Cow dung may be placed
on the infant's cord to stop the bleeding, and therefore
tetanus is not uncommon. Twins are bad luck to economically
depressed people and therefore one child may be neglected or
even killed. Our culture abhors such behavior, yet our infant mortality rate is high (19.8 for 1970). We provide
our own equivalent of cow dung - Thalidomide to pregnant
mothers resulting in armless children is one we know about.
Synthetic estrogens to stop uterine bleeding consequently

giving rise to vaginal carcinomas in the adolescent daughters
fifteen to twenty years later - is another.[4]

Functionally, the breast is gradually becoming a ves-
tigial organ. Many women are "dried up" immediately post-
partum with some form of estrogen preparation - sometimes
even without their permission. During pregnancy and immediately after, the breast becomes the obstetrician's problem.
When breast abcesses develop or lumps are palpated it belongs
to the surgeon. The infant hardly ever sees the breast. In
all other mammals it belongs to the newborn - not so in our
"cultured" human society.

Primitive societies have a lot to learn from us and
strangely enough we can learn something from them. The
medicine-man "throws the bones" for his patient. "There is
a tall man", he says. "Yes", answers the patient, "it is
my husband." The bones are thrown again. "He is angry."
"Yes - he is angry because I cannot give him a child." The
medicine-man takes his time. Slowly, he obtains the history
while he gains the patient's confidence. Then he prescribes
an herb. If it works, he gets paid. If not, he doesn't. In
our society, the patient pays whichever way it goes!

FOLKLORE AND OBSTETRICS

Folklore in many parts is well founded. Rhymes and
fairy tales give insight into sensible practices. The story
of Rapunzel is in fact one of these. Here the pregnant

mother, as she grew paler and weaker, craved greens growing
in the witch's garden. This evidently supplied her folate
needs for she became strong and well. In some African tribes,
eating eggs and even drinking milk is considered harmful to
the unborn infant.[7] These women gauge their stage of gestation by the color of the breast secretion expressed.

    During pregnancy folklore, suspicion and fear of the
unknown exists at all socioeconomic levels and in all parts
of the world. Many of these practices affect the fetus
during growth and development and result in serious consequences. Malnutrition in the mother may affect intelligence
and even brain development in the fetus.[5]

RITUALS, ROUTINES

    Routine post-operative gastric suction for all abdominal
cases is still a ritual in many hospitals.[8] Skin preparations may be necessary to provide surgical access. Seropian
and Reynolds[6] found a 5.6% infection rate after shaving the
skin compared to 0.6% when no shave was carried out. The
infection rate was 3.1% if shaving was carried out immediately
before the operation, but rose to 20% if performed 24 hours
or more before surgery because of minor infections in nicked
and abraded skin after shaving. The routine cleansing of the
skin prior to giving an injection or pulling blood has been
shown to be of little value but is still practiced.[2] In
short, rituals should be periodically reexamined and evaluated.

REFERENCES

1.   Bradley RA: Husband-Coached Childbirth. New York,
     Harper & Row, 1965

2.   Dann TC: Routine skin preparation before injection.
     Lancet 2:96, 1969

3.   Dick-Read G: Childbirth without Fear. Second edition.
     New York, Harper & Row, 1960

4.   Herbst AL, Ulfelder H, Poskanzer DC: Adenocarcinoma
     of the vagina: Association of maternal stilboestrol
     therapy with tumor appearance in young women. New
     Eng J Med 284:878, 1971

5.   Nutrition and the developing brain. Lancet 2:1349,
     1972 (Editorial)

6.   Seropian R, Reynolds BM: Sterilization of the skin.
     Amer Jour of Surgery 121:251, 1971

7.   Simons WH: Eat Not This Flesh. Madison, University
     of Wisconsin Press, 1961

8.   Surgical rituals. BMJ   3:543, 1972 (Editorial)

9.   Williams CD, Jelliffe DB: Mother and Child Health:
     Delivering the Services. New York, Oxford University
     Press, 1972

CHAPTER 3

Obstetrics

LUIS SALDANA and NAOMI BAUMSLAG

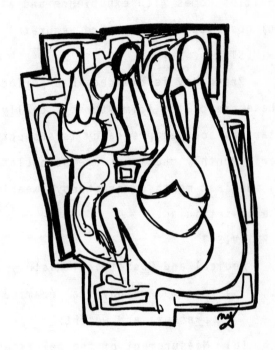

PRENATAL CARE

PRENATAL CARE MAY be defined as the supervision
and care of the pregnant and parturient woman to
ensure that she has a pregnancy and later a labor with the
least possible risk and fear, and gives birth to a living
child which she will be fit to nurture.

Watchful waiting, emotional support and parental education are most important during this time. During pregnancy, certain guidelines are used to monitor basic levels and to spot deviations from the normal. The ability to spot abnormalities comes with experience and also with constant, careful observations which are accurately documented.

TRIMESTER

Pregnancy is divided into periods of three months. These are called trimesters. Ideally, prenatal visits should start as soon as pregnancy is suspected in the first trimester. Monthly check-ups are scheduled throughout pregnancy. In the last month of pregnancy, weekly visits are made to the obstetrician.

FIRST VISIT

1. Medical and Obstetrical History
2. (a) A complete physical examination including blood pressure and weight.
    (b) Measurement of the pelvis and pelvic examination.
    (c) Breasts
    (d) Special attention to nutritional state
3. Laboratory Tests
    (a) Blood group and type Rh A B O
        (1) Hemoglobin and Hematocrit
    (b) Serology - Venereal Disease (VDRL)
    (c) Urine for protein, sugar and cellular content

OBSTETRICAL HISTORY

A good obstetrical history provides invaluable information. In addition to a detailed general history, special note is made of the following:

1. Attitude

    Determine the patient's attitude to the pregnancy. In successive visits look for changes such as depression, fatigue, irritability.

2. Age

    Complications increase with increase in age; for example, high blood pressure, diabetes, mongolism in offspring. Mongolism was formerly thought to occur in "old" women only, but recent evidence suggests the mothers of mongols may also age prematurely.

3. Gravida

    Total number of pregnancies that patient has including the present pregnancy, abortions, premature and stillbirths. Primigravid - 1st pregnancy. Young women bearing their first infant have a higher incidence of complications in pregnancy and labor and also a higher stillborn and prematurity rate.

4. Para

    The number of viable pregnancies (over 20 weeks or over 500 gm weight) that the patient has delivered in the past. Usually one less than gravida unless an abortion

has occurred. Stillborns and premature births are included.

5. Multiple Pregnancy

Pregnancies in which there are more than one fetus
(twins, quads) are more prone to complications, anemia,
prematurity, toxemia. Often there is a family history
that alerts. Women with high parity also have a higher
incidence of multiple pregnancies.

6. Abortions

The number of nonviable pregnancies in the past (under
20 weeks gestation or 500 gm in weight).

7. LMP

Last date of normal menstrual period that the patient
menstruated (the patient will often give the date of
the 1st period that they missed. However, only 20 percent of females can tell you exactly the LMP to the
day).

8. EDC ((Expected date of confinement)[12]

This is calculated if patient is pregnant by subtracting
3 months from the date of the first day of the LMP and
to this add 7 days, e.g. LMP (1st day) July 7. Sub-
tract 3 months - April 7; add 7 days - April 14 - EDC.
This is for a 28 day cycle. For a 35 day cycle add 7
days more, for a 25 day menstrual cycle substract 3
days. The error of this estimation can be two weeks

late or two weeks early. The latter mistake is appreciated; the former is not! Of course, if the LMP is
inaccurate, then this figure will be wrong. The patient
should be told that this is only an approximation.

9.   Quickening

This is a subjective feeling of fetal movements by the
patient. By itself it is not a true sign of pregnancy
as it can be caused by the movements of a fibroid on a
pedicle or bowel peristalsis or uterine contractions
known as Braxton Hicks contractions. Quickening usually
occurs in the 20th week of pregnancy.

PREGNANCY

Early Symptoms

1.   Amenorrhea - missed menstruation periods

2.   Early morning sickness

3.   Breast tenderness

4.   Loss of waist line, clothes don't fit as they used to

Early Signs

1.   Dilatation of superficial veins of breast 6-8th week.
      One of the most readily detected signs.

2.   Blueish discoloration of vagina and cervix

3.   Uterine softening and enlargement - progressive

4.   Pulsation in lateral fornices due to dilation and tor-
      tuosity of uterine arteries - easily detectable and a
      reliable sign.

5.   Hyperpigmentation: areola - around nipples; chloasma -
      facial mask; linea nigra - abdominal mid-line marking

<u>Biological Test</u>[7]

The best is the Latex flocculation "slide test". Gra-
videx (Ortho) Test is one frequently used. Results depend
on following instructions: blood and protein in urine can
affect results, presence of a trace of detergent in equipment used may cause false results. Test depends on HCG
(human chorionic gonadotrophin) which is significantly raised
one week after the first missed period and reaches peak at
the 10th week. (L.H. - luteinizing hormone in premenopausal
women may result in a false positive test). There are many
other causes of false positives or false negatives and the
literature should be consulted. The absence of flocculation
is interpreted as a positive test and is indicative of pregnancy almost invariably.

The following symptoms and signs necessitate admission
when physical findings indicate:

1.   <u>Excessive vomiting</u> - the patient may become dehydrated.

2.   <u>Bleeding</u> - compare blood loss to a normal period and
      ask how many pads are used and if clots have been
      passed.

      a.   Many patients will have spotting in the presence
            of severe vaginitis. However, it is wise to in-
            vestigate vaginal bleeding regardless of the

probable cause.

b. A first trimester abortion occurs in about 15% of
    all pregnancies.

c. Ectopic pregnancy occurs in 1/200 pregnancies
    (ectopic = not in the endometrium).

d. Placenta Praevia (placenta over cervix) occurs in
    the third trimester. The patient is <u>not</u> to be
    examined, but admit for evaluation of the bleeding.
    Type and cross match compatible blood. Expectant
    treatment if fetus has not reached maturity. Pla-
    cental scan or ultrasound for diagnosis. Excessive
    bleeding is an indication for Cesarean Section.
    Double set-up exam if fetus is over 37 weeks or
    the fetal weight is over 2500 grams.

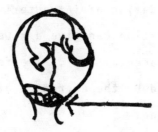

Placenta Praevia
(placenta is first)

e. Abruptio placenta - board-like, tender abdomen due
    to premature separation of the placenta. Check co-
    agulation and fibrinogen. Type and cross match
    blood. If the fetus is viable a Cesarean Section
    may be necessary.

3. <u>Abdominal Pain</u> - occurs in an ectopic pregnancy espe-
    cially if an adnexal mass is present. Pain also is
    present in abortions or premature labor. Abortion
    occurs more frequently than ectopic or premature labor.
    If there is abdominal pain, be sure an exact descrip-
    tion is made; duration, severity, type and interval of
    the pains. R/o urinary tract infection, APPENDICITIS.

4. <u>Draining amniotic fluid</u> - Ruptured membranes lead to
    premature labor or amnionitis which pose a fetal hazard

5. <u>Hypertension, Diabetes and Renal Disease</u> are indication
    for admission in order to evaluate the maternal state.
    Intrauterine growth retardation and antepartum death
    are definite risks in these conditions. Serial sono-
    graphic measurements of the biparietal diameter can be
    used to detect retardation of intrauterine growth.
    Serial estrogen excretion can give a clue to the well-
    being of the feto-placental unit. The feto-placental
    unit can be evaluated by the excretion of estrogen
    (estriol) in the urine.

6. <u>Convulsions</u> - especially due to toxemia of pregnancy.
AVOID X-RAYS AND ALL DRUGS IN THE FIRST THREE MONTHS OF
AMENORRHEA WHEN ORGANOGENESIS IS OCCURRING.[19]
PHYSICAL EXAMINATION
    Remember to be tactful, polite and promote <u>privacy</u>.
Not many women like to be examined as if they were strippers

Cover the exposed parts not being examined. A female atten-
dant's presence is advisable during the examination. Always
tell the mother what progress she is making and if you are
going to do a pelvic, explain this and tell her what to
expect.

General Examination

The facial expression of the patient, her posture and
the way she behaves can tell you a lot about her attitude to
the pregnancy. During the routine physical exam pay special
attention to:

B.P. (Blood pressure)	Breasts
Weight	Abdomen
Teeth	Pelvic
Heart	Legs for varicosities and edema
Lungs	Anemia

B.P.

Chart the B.P. throughout pregnancy. A baseline level is
extremely important, so see that the patient is as relaxed
as possible. Hypertension predisposes to complications in
pregnancy, but meticulous care can save the baby of a hypertensive mother. A rise of systolic pressure over 140 mm of
mercury and diastolic above 90 mm should alert one to pre-
eclampsia.

Edema

Check for swelling (edema) of extremities and presacral edema.
Remember that tight stockings or girdles may impede venous
return and cause edema. Albuminuria may require admission

to prevent toxemia espeically if a low sodium diet and bed rest fail to stem this. Prophyllactic diuretics <u>do not</u> prevent the occurrence of pre-eclampsia.[10]

Weight

Chart the weight also. A weight gain of more than 5 lb/month or 2 lb/week is abnormal.

Teeth

The mother's teeth should be checked. Fluoride may be needed for dental nutrition and skeletal growth in the fetus.

Breasts

Look at the nipples, secretions, vascularity. Note the comparative size of both breasts. Feel for texture, irregularity and masses.

Abdomen

1. Feel

    Leopold's manoeuvers -

    a. Palpate the abdomen to ascertain which part of the fetus occupies the fundus.

    b. Ascertain the position of fetal back and small parts.

    c. Palpate the presenting part to determine if it is <u>cephalic</u> or <u>breech</u>.

    d. Is the head engaged, i.e. too low to ballot abdominally?

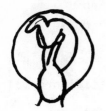 Vertex   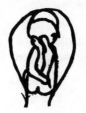 Breech

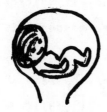 Transverse lie

2.   Measure the height of the uterus in centimeters.[1]
     Figure below gives a very rough guide to the normal
     rate of growth.

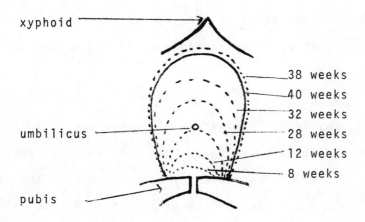

Stops growing in: 1. missed abortion

2. fetal death

Growth faster than normal: 1. twins - multiple pregna

2. hydatidiform moles

3.   Listen - Fetal heart (F.H.) is heard usually around the
     20th week (ask the patient if quickening has been felt)
     The position of fetal heart sounds is variable. Usuall
     in a vertex (head) presentation, which is by far the
     commonest, it is heard on the same side as the fetal
     back and below the maternal umbilicus. The fetal heart
     rate is fast, about 140 beats per minute. Compare this
     with the normal adult pulse rate of 70 beats per minute
     If "life" is felt, i.e. fetal movements, the F.H. shoul
     be there. In case of doubt Doptone can be used to de-
     tect the fetal heart.

4.   Estimate the fetal weight: Muscle tone, abdominal size
     the amount of amniotic fluid - all influence the esti-
     mate.

Pelvic Examination

     This should be done with maximum privacy. Have a nurse
with you and don't take longer than necessary. Reassure the
patient. If a metal speculum is used, make sure that it is
warm! Don't lubricate the speculum with jelly, use water.

1.   Vulva - Examine, see if there is any swelling, discharg
     or ulcers.

2.   Urethra - Milk for a discharge.

3.   Vagina - Look for a discharge and note color, odor and
     microscopic appearance.

COMMON DISCHARGES: Discharges are common in the last trimester of pregnancy - if associated with pruritius (itching)
the mother may be very uncomfortable. Make a smear and try
to identify the organism.

1.   Yellow to greenish - gonorrhea - intra-cellular gram
     negative cocci. Culture in Thayer-Martin medium.

2.   White curd-like - moniliasis - mycelia in KOH (potassium
     hydroxide on slide)

3.   Yellow-green, foul-smelling - trichomonas - flagellates
     (saline on slide)

4.   Tan color - bacteria

Lab Tests

     The most common anemia in pregnancy is iron deficiency
anemia. A low hematocrit (under 35), or hemoglobin below
11 gm %, may alert one to this problem. However, in pregnancy the plasma volume increases up to 40 percent, causing
a dilutional "anemia". There is a compensatory rise in rbc
volume of 400 cc which is dependent on an adequate iron intake. A less common anemia is due to folic acid deficiency.
The supplementation of folic acid and iron during pregnancy
is routine in many centers. The need for supplementation is
due to increased demands in pregnancy by the growing fetus.

Blood should be checked for type: Rh positive blood is present in 85 percent, and Rh negative blood is found in 15 percent of women. In Rh negative women, precautions are taken to prevent erythroblastosis fetalis and Rh antibody titres are checked at 28, 32, 36 and 38 weeks. If positive at 1:64 or over, amniocentesis should be performed. Schulman and others have set guide lines for management of these cases according to results of spectrophotometric examination of amniotic fluid. Urine is checked for sugar and protein in order to detect diabetes and renal disease. Diabetes mellitus is difficult to define but a single positive urine test or a single raised blood sugar does not necessarily mean the patient is diabetic. Glycosuria is common in pregnancy. Where urinary tract infections are suspected, the urine is sent for culture and urinalysis. Stools should be examined for color (patients on iron tablets have stools that are blackish in color, ferrous sulphide) and for parasites.

Serology must also be checked. Congenital syphilis carries not only social stigmata but also debilitatory consequences for the child.

General Advice

Provide relevant educational material and check to see if there are any questions.

Unless it is uncomfortable or causes bleeding, there is no reason why a pregnant woman can't have intercourse until she delivers.

Introduce her to your partner or your substitute in
case you are away at the time of delivery.

LABOR

As it implies, it is hard work.

Labor usually starts at 38 weeks after conception or
40 weeks after the last menstrual period. It begins when
the cervix starts to dilate and painful contractions appear.

1st Stage

Begins with true labor contractions which are usually
painful and ends with complete dilatation of the cervix and
may last from 2 to 16 hours or more. Initially they are
10-15 minutes apart, and later 2 minutes apart; sometimes
lasting 30-35 seconds early in labor and then increasing to
90 seconds. Time the duration of the contractions and the
interval between them. Remember that primigravidas having
"pains" every 5 minutes should come in at that stage. In
multiparas, patients having contractions at ten minute intervals should come in as they often have very short labor.

The first stage can be divided into a latent and an
active phase. The cervical dilatation can be estimated by
comparing the transverse diameter of the cervix as felt by
2 fingers with a premeasured plastic cervical mold. As experience is gained, the estimate of cervical dilatation becomes easier. The dividing point is 4 cms dilatation. This

can be plotted as illustrated with the dotted line repre-
senting the latent phase.[16,17]

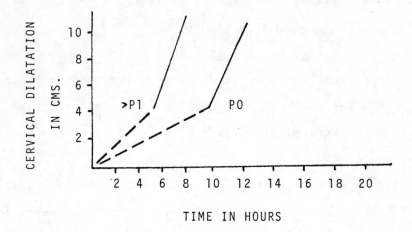

TIME IN HOURS

These curves represent the <u>mean</u> duration of the latent and
active phase of labor for nulliparous (PO) and multiparous
(Pl) patients. Since these represent mean duration, two
standard deviations can still be normal. The active phase
should not be prolonged over 4 hours although the latent
phase shows great variability (2-18 hours). Any deviation
should cause concern and prompt the obstetrician to seek a
reason for it. X-ray pelvimetry and evaluation of the uterine contractions are necessary. Unfortunately there is no
accurate way of determining the fetal size which is probably
the most significant variable.

     In the last decade intrauterine electronic (Hon) and
biochemical fetal monitoring have been introduced.[8] This has

revolutionized the management of high-risk patients in labor.
It is possible to record the fetal heart rate (FHR) and the
uterine contractions continuously.[8,14] Certain abnormalities
in the FHR are indications for fetal blood analysis to detect
hypoxia.[9] This affords the obstetrician complete evaluation
of the fetal state. In addition, the frequency and intensity of uterine contractions can be evaluated. Great ad-
vances have also been made in intrauterine fetal monitoring
during labor which is beneficial in high-risk cases of diabetes mellitus, hypertension and post-maturity.

2nd Stage

Complete dilatation of cervix to expulsion of baby.

DELIVERY

The delivery may be supervised without any drugs, anesthesia or episiotomy (natural childbirth) or may be assisted
with drugs and instruments.

Emotional support is essential during labor. In addition, it has become customary to administer sedatives and
analgesics to women in labor to allow them to relax between
contractions.

The techniques used for pain relief in labor are many
and varied.

1.   Analgesia

Used in first stage; reduces pain. Usually demerol
plus an antiemetic or tranquilizer. Used in excess,

it depresses respiration of the fetus.

2. Anesthesia

    a. General anesthesia is available (fluothane and
        Nitrous oxide); used early in the 2nd stage of
        labor. If a generous (50%) oxygen mixture is
        used, the fetus is rarely depressed.

    b. Conduction anesthesia eliminates or reduces
        "bearing down" sensation.

        1. Spinal (saddle block)

        2. Epidural, caudal or lumbar (used in the active
           phase)

        3. Pudendal block (late labor)

Blood absorption and trans-placental transfer of Lido-
caine or carbocaine can cause fetal or neonatal depression
due to apnea and cardiac arrest.

When the head appears at the vulva, an episiotomy is
commonly performed and is mandatory in primips. This may be
a medio-lateral or less desirably a midline incision of the
perineum: 1. to prevent uncontrolled tears or lacerations,
2. because straight incisions in a controlled direction
heal more rapidly and are more easily sutured, 3. to prevent damage to the newborn. Episiotomy repair is often performed under a local pudendal block.

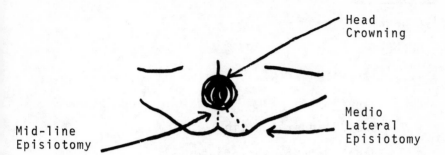

Head
Crowning

Medio
Lateral
Episiotomy

Mid-line
Episiotomy

3rd Stage

1)   Placental separation

2)   Placental expulsion

Make sure that the uterus is empty, firm and contracted.
Check to see that the placenta is complete and that all the
cotyledons are present. A full bladder frequently contri-
butes to post partum hemorrhage therefore make sure the bladder is empty. Putting baby to the breast causes uterine contractions. Ergotrate or oxytocin may be given to stop utero-
placental bleeding. In cases of post-partum hemorrhage, a
thorough examination of the uterine cavity, cervix, vagina
and episiotomy is essential. Retained placental fragments,
cervical and vaginal tears are common causes of post-partum
hemorrhage. Uterine rupture and episiotomy hematomas will
cause blood loss.

After Delivery (Post Partum)

Daily check:

A. Mother

1. Vital signs

2. Breasts

3. Bowel/bladder function

4. Fundal height (top of uterus)

5. Perineum (stitches). Lochia - during the puer-
peral period (6 week period following the birth
of infant) there is usually some discharge. In
the first two weeks it is usually red to brownish
in color. After 2 weeks it becomes whitish.

6. Extremities

7. Rest

B. Baby

1. Cord

2. Circumcision

3. Feeding

4. Diapers

5. Weight

BEFORE THE MOTHER AND BABY LEAVE THE HOSPITAL, TAKE TIME TO
REINFORCE THE FUNDAMENTALS IN INFANT CARE SUCH AS BATHING,
FEEDING AND ACCIDENT PREVENTION FACTS THAT THE MOTHER
SHOULD HAVE BECOME FAMILIAR WITH PRENATALLY.

FAMILY PLANNING

The consumer decides, the physician can only make suggestions and give information. Find out if some form of family planning is intended, and if so, what type. I.U.D.'s (intrauterine devices) are best inserted during the menses or within 6 weeks post partum. Menses usually resumes 6 to 8 weeks after delivery if not breast feeding. If breast feeding, menses may be delayed but birth control is still necessary.

A sensible presentation of available types of contraception should be made. Draw attention to various advantages and disadvantages and invite questions. Most of all, since it is up to the patient, let her make the decision. Couples usually choose the method of brith control that is the most natural and most comfortable for them.

PLANNED PARENTHOOD[2,4,15]

Sexual taboos, social or class attitudes and legal implications of illegitimate offspring all influence sexual relationships. In the transplant age there is liberalization of sexual restraint prior to marriage and altered attitude to unplanned families. There are more than nine million women on the "pill" in this country. In addition, legalization of abortion by the Supreme Court of the United States is further evidence of changing attitudes to pregnancy. No longer does a woman have to carry an unwanted baby. The

middle class and rich have always been able to restrict
family size or do something about it. Attempts are being
made to make it more available to other groups. Why a woman
should have to carry, deliver and then rear an unwanted
child is a question now being asked since it may mean suffering for the mother, the child, and later society. The
discovery of prostaglandins may provide abortions more easily
than surgical procedures currently available. They may even
be used for producing expulsion of the fetus at a required
time. Amniocentesis has been developed to detect fetal abnormalities in diseases of genetic origin.[3] The procedure
itself is not without risk - bleeding and infection can
occur. The problems of, and indications for, abortion in
such cases are not always clear cut and even in the best
hands, the risk of aborting a perfectly formed fetus exists.[1]

Organized efforts are being made to help reduce family
size by conscientious planning. In many parts of the world,
such as India, men are suspicious of their wives' morality
and would rather be sterilized themselves than to have
their wives "sexually free". The lure of contraception to
people of some cultural groups is negligible. For instance
in tribal Africa, a man's wealth is obtained by marrying
off his daughters in exchange for cattle (labolo) and children are important as a source of labor. For most countries
the cost, on a national basis, would be prohibitive if the

pill were used and the I.U.D. insertion requires skilled
manpower.

I.   THE PILL (Oral Contraceptives)

As yet there is no ideal method of contraception. Currently, oral contraceptives are most frequently used. These
are usually a combination of estrogen and progesterone to
inhibit ovulation. The main action is to inhibit the hypo-
thalamus from releasing FSH and/or LH releasing factors and
so the ovary receives no stimulus for the growth and development of the graafian follicle. In addition, there is an alteration of the viscosity of cervical secretion rendering
entry of the sperm into the uterine cavity more difficult.
Although this method is almost 100% effective, a dedicated
degree of motivation and the ability to follow instructions
are essential.

Absolute Contraindications to Birth Control Pills are:

1.   Patients with a history of phlebitis, or pulmonary
      embolism

2.   Hypertensives, especially of renal origin

3.   Cancer of the breast and pelvic organs

4.   Pregnancy

Many obstetricians do not consider age a contraindication to the use of the birth control pill. One must keep in
mind that contraindications to the use of birth control pills
are frequently also contraindications to pregnancy. In these

women surgical sterilization should seriously be considered. Rheumatic heart disease may also be a contraindication because of the risk of mural thrombi. Pregnancy may also be contraindicated in females known to have rheumatic carditis. An I.U.D. would be advisable for them. Headaches are not an absolute contraindication to the pill, and patients may take them as long as their headaches do not become worse. However, when headaches appear while on the pill, discontinue them for that reason.

It must be remembered that this is not a physiological process and that the menstrual cycle can be adjusted to whatever intervals are required by adjusting the therapy.

Today we aim at the lowest effective estrogen dosage which is 50 micrograms. Furthermore, it is advisable for a woman who wants to have more children to stop every two years for a short period so as to allow the menstrual cycle to revert for 2 or 3 cycles. During this period she must either not have intercourse or must use the diaphragm, condom or jelly if she does not want to become pregnant.

Instructions to Patients:

1.   Watch out for:

     a.   Severe leg cramps

     b.   Severe headaches or dizzy spells

     c.   Blurred vision

     d.   Chest pain

2. During the first two weeks on oral contraceptives, use
    another method of birth control as well.

3. Take your pill at the same time each day - less nausea
    if taken at night.

4. If you have continued spotting or other problems, con-
    sult your obstetrician or clinic doctor.

NOTE: Continued spotting must be investigated and a D & C
should be performed in these cases to rule out polyps or
encometrial cancer.

II. INTRAUTERINE DEVICE

This is an old method of contraception. It was used by
Arabian camel drivers who placed a stone in the reproductive
canals of camels to prevent pregnancy during caravans. There
are many types available. They are steel or polyethelene
foreign bodies which are inserted into the uterus and usually
have nylon "tail" (strings) which can be felt by the patient
at the cervical os.

Coil   Lippes   Dalcon
              Loop   Shield

This is introduced either at the time of the period, (as it may cause bleeding) or at the three week post partum check up. The former time is preferable. At these times one can be reasonably sure that the patient is not pregnant and the cervical canal is more patent. Immediate post partum insertion has an expulsion rate of 3% which is not prohibitively high. The possible mechanisms of action of the I.U.D. are:

1. Macrophage foreign body reaction with digestion of sperms and/or the fertilized egg.

2. Rapid transit of ova (not likely)

This method has an effectiveness of 98% if not expelled. It does not require any patient motivation or extensive instructions to the patient.

The disadvantages of the I.U.D. are:

1. Expulsion which varies with both the type of device and the number of children that the patient has delivered.

2. The I.U.D. may become embedded under the endometrium and then is very difficult to remove. Very rarely it erodes the uterine wall and perforates.

3. Chronic pelvic infection may be aggravated especially with metallic devices.

4. Excess menstrual flow may occur and/or may be associated with severe cramps. The patient may demand removal.

Instructions to Patients:

Men do not usually feel the strings during intercourse.
The first menstrual period may be heavier than normal.
Cramps may occur during the first 24 hours. However if
severe, contact your doctor. Feel for the I.U.D. strings
weekly during the first month and especially after the first
menstrual period. Contact the doctor if (1) no strings are
found (2) if a hard mass or the plastic of the I.U.D. is at
the cervical os. If the strings are not visible when
the patient returns to the clinic, insert a uterine sound
to feel for the I.U.D. and measure the uterine cavity. If
the I.U.D. (foreign-body sensation) is felt with sound and
the uterine cavity is no larger than usual, nothing else
need be done. If the I.U.D. cannot be felt, then the patient
should be scheduled for a hysterosalpingogram after a pregnancy test. Prior to a hystersalpingogram a flat plate is
done. If it fails to reveal the I.U.D. in the abdomen or
pelvis, inadvertent expulsion is the diagnosis. If the
I.U.D. is revealed, then a hysterosalpingogram will outline
the uterine cavity and the exact relation of the I.U.D. to
the uterus can be ascertained. A laparotomy or a colpotomy
is then performed to retrieve it.

III. DIAPHRAGM

This is a rubber shield which has to be fitted according
to vaginal size by a physician. Its effectiveness is around

80-90% depending on the user. It acts as a mechanical block of sperms. Requires high motivation on the part of the patient. In some instances, this method is used periodically or on "danger" days.

Instructions to Patients:

Demonstrate how to insert and check that the diaphragm is in the correct position. Teach the patient how to feel the cervix through the diaphragm. Use charts and models to help her understand.

Explain that the correct size is the largest size worn without discomfort during intercourse. It must be used together with a spermicidal jelly or foam. Place the diaphragm in position not more than 6-8 hours before intercourse and remove it 8-16 hours after.

The diaphragm must be washed with soap and water, rinsed, dried and coated with talcum powder or corn starch. Check regularly for defects.

IV. CONDOMS (Rubbers)

This is an effective method and is especially useful in teenagers who have sporadic or infrequent intercourse. This method substantially reduces the risk of venereal disease in high school and college populations.

Instructions to Patients:

1. Use a lubricated condom as it has less tendency to tear. If a condom is used more than once, vaseline should not

be used as it decomposes the rubber. Heat also has the
same effect.

2.   During removal of the penis from the vagina, the male
must hold the rim of the condom to avoid leakage or
spillage. Also remove soon after ejaculation.

3.   Female can be encouraged to put the condom on for the
male as part of the loveplay.

4.   Lambskin type is the best.

V.   RHYTHM

This requires high motivation and should be used with
abstinence as it is not as effective as the above methods.
Its usefulness is increased if ovulation time is checked
with basal body temperature. Contraindicated in women with
irregular menses.

VI. SURGICAL METHODS

Female

Tubal Resection

    1.   Bilateral salpingectomy: Performed post partum
or 6 weeks after delivery and consists of removing
both fallopian tubes. Very effective.

    2.   Partial salpingectomy

        a.   Resection of the isthmic portion and the
burial of the proximal end of tube into
the myometrium by a suture.

    b.   Ligation and resection of isthmic portion
of tube.

In many hospitals a quota system for Tubal Ligation exists. This is based on the age of the mother x the number of children = number of points. The usual number of points is 120 plus and then she still may have to wait as only a certain number are performed each week.

It must be noted that permission of the husband is mandatory in some states for a tubal ligation unless legally separated. In unmarried women, this is not required. It is somewhat ironic that a woman may give permission for a major operation such as a hysterectomy, yet for a tubal ligation which is a minor procedure, the husband's consent is required at some medical centers. Men on the other hand do not need their wives' written approval for a vasectomy.

Note: The American College of Obstetricians and Gynecologists do not require the husband's permission for tubal ligation.

Male

Vasectomy is the resection of the testicular portion of the vas deferens. This is done as an office procedure under local anesthesia. Due to the pool of sperms in the seminal vesicles, proximal vas and the prostate gland postoperatively the tenth or eleventh ejaculate should be examined.

               . . . .

There is more to obstetrics than labor and delivery. Obstetricians and nurse-midwives offer continuity care. They provide family planning, patient education, and immediate newborn care. The family is to be viewed as a whole and treated as an entity.

Many obstetricians have come to realize that mid-wives or physician technicians can perform most of the uncomplicated deliveries with the aid and support of the husband. This frees the obstetrician to give better care to the patients showing prenatal or intra-partum complications.

REFERENCES

1. Beazley JM, Underhill RA: Fallacy of the fundal height.
    Brit Med J 4:404, 1970

2. Contraceptive Technology. Emory University Family
    Planning Program, 1972

3. Edwards JH: Uses of amniocentesis. Lancet 1:608, 1970

4. Feingold A, Cherniak D: Birth Control Handbook. Quebec
    McGill University, 1969

5. Greenhill J: Obstetrics. Philadelphia, Saunders, 1965

6. Williams JW: Obstetrics. Fourteenth edition by LM
    Hellman, JA Pritchard. New York, Appleton-Century-
    Crofts, 1971

7. Hibbard BM: Pregnancy diagnosis. Brit Med J 1:593,
    1971

8. Hon EH: Electronic evaluation of the fetal heart rate.
    Amer J Obstet Gynec 75:1215, 1958

9. Hon EH: Observations on 'pathologic' fetal bradicardia.
    Amer J Obstet Gynec 77:1084, 1959

10. Kraus GW, Marchese JR, Yen SSC: Prophyllactic use of
    hydrochlorothiazide in pregnancy. JAMA 198:1150, 1966

11. Lappe M, Gustafson JM, Roblin R: Ethical and social
    issues in screening for genetic disease. New Eng J
    Med 286:1129, 1972

12. Length of gestation. Brit Med J 4:582, 1972. (Editoria

13. Leonard CO, Chase GN, Childs B: Genetic counseling:
    A consumer's view. New Eng J Med 287:433, 1972

14. Paul RH, Hon EH: A clinical fetal monitor. Obstet
    Gynec 35:161, 1970

15. Peel J, Potts D: Textbook of Contraceptive Practice.
    Cambridge, Cambridge University Press, 1969

16. Schulman H, Ledger W: Practical application of the
    graphic portrayal of labor. Obstet Gynec 23:442, 1964

17.   Schulman H: Prolonged and abnormal labor. Amer J
      Obstet Gynec 95:732, 1966

18.   Schulman H, Mann L, Hayashi TT: The Rh sensitized
      pregnant woman. JAMA 196:177, 1966

19.   Stewart AM, Kneale GW: Age-distribution of cancers
      caused by obstetric x-rays and their relevance to cancer
      latent periods. Lancet 2:4, 1970

CHAPTER 4

Pediatrics

LOUISE RAUH, NAOMI BAUMSLAG,
and CLARICE REID

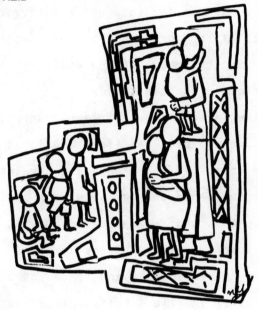

A CHILD'S HEALTH cannot be viewed in isolation.

The impact of both the internal and external environment has far reaching effects. The malnourished mother
may deprive her infant of certain essentials. Undernourished
mothers may give birth prematurely to infants of low birth
weight. Mercury and lead poisoning have occurred in utero
with resultant toxic effects on the newborn. Infections
such as syphilis, gonorrhea, toxoplasmosis, cytomegalic

77

inclusion disease, and rubella can all have serious impact
on the fetus. Many deficiencies and infections have been
linked with epilepsy, diabetes, hyperkinetic children, and
children with mental retardation. The drugs used during
pregnancy, such as thalidomides and terramycins can affect
the health of the infant and mother;[13] LSD may produce chro-
mosomal damage. Trauma during delivery also results in
maimed or brain-damaged children.

As the infant enters his environment, the interplay of
factors such as love, handling, feeding and someone talking
or making sounds affect growth and development. Children
from damp overcrowded homes with poor hygiene are more prone
to tuberculosis and rheumatic fever. The poor, being more
crowded, tend to get infections earlier. Richer children
are usually more isolated and are exposed to infectious
diseases later in life. Poliomyelitis was more common in
children of wealthier backgrounds who had not had any chance
to build up an immunity.

Parents influence behavior, speech and outlook. Unmarried mothers often see the same set of problems early in
their daughters. If for example sodomy is practiced in a
family, it will be accepted as "normal" by the offspring.[7]
Burns may be commonplace where cooking is done over an open
fire; trichinosis affects families who eat uncooked meat.
Pinworm (seat worm) is a familial infestation and, therefore,

all the members of a family may be in need of medical treatment.

Growth patterns, speech, weight, height, motor activities
and psychological development are all influenced markedly
by social and cultural factors.[5] The old Japanese custom of
swaddling babies resulted in stunting of infants. African
mothers carry their babies on their backs without supporting
the baby's head. Caucasians have a fear that the baby's
head will be damaged if the baby is not supported when held
up. The playfulness of the family or its obsessiveness with
routines all have their impact on the growth of a happy
healthy child. To know a child one must know the family,
the home and the neighborhood. This is even more essential
for the handicapped and chronically ill children. It is not
sufficient to examine the child and then prescribe medicine.
Each situation requires consideration of all the operative
factors. For example, if a family has osteogenesis imperfecta it is not enough to treat the fractures and describe
the family tree. A protective school environment, not always
easy to find, will have to be sought for some children. A
child with rheumatic fever needs more than daily prophylactic
penicillin; the home must not be damp, good food should be
provided and adequate or special education may be needed.
The psychological effects of illness should be compensated
as best as possible.[11] Symptoms of illness affect the

entire family and put unusual stresses on the individual
members.

THE RELATIONSHIP BETWEEN THE FAMILY AND THE DOCTOR

The doctor should be warm and friendly but not "familiar"
with members of the family since resentment, lack of cooperation and even hostility may result. In the case of an
"unmarried mother" check with her as to how she desires to
be addressed. It is unwise to take sides in family fights,
give gifts or money as this will only produce a sense of
obligation and may distort the relationship but won't solve
the problems.

If a question cannot be answered or the diagnosis is
uncertain, it is best to say so and then try to find someone
who has the information. The family should
be informed of any tests that may
have to be done and the rationale
for the tests explained in a
clear and simple manner without using ill-understood
medical terminology. Questions should be encouraged.
To obtain the trust of the
family it is essential to be
honest and forthright. Blunt-
ness should be avoided. For

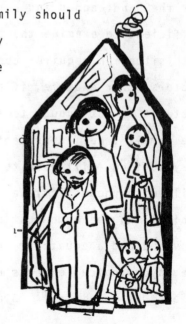

example, don't say, "Your child will be blind if an operation is not done!" Instead tell the parents that the eye-
sight is poor, that there has been damage to the cornea and
that an operation should be performed as soon as can be
arranged, but do not leave the anxious parents nervously
guessing. Praise should be freely given where it is indicated. It is not one's intent to produce a clinging family,
but rather to encourage independence while assuring that the
doctor is available for consultation or re-examination when
needed.

Appointments should be kept but if there is an unavoid-
albe delay, the patient and the parent need to be told about
it. It is unfair to keep an anxious mother with one or more
irritable children waiting endlessly. If necessary, schedule
another appointment.

Following the examination, thank both mother and child
for their cooperation. This is an important point, for
sometimes what passes for normal behavior as far as the doctor is concerned, is considered as "bad" behavior by the
parent. Subsequent scolding at home may put a barrier between child and doctor.

In Haggerty's study[6] phone calls constitute at least
12% of pediatric practice. In some practices this figure
is considerably higher. If a parent calls repeatedly, the
doctor should not automatically react negatively and regard

the parent as a pest. The phone calls may be cries for help
or symptomatic of some deeper underlying family problems.

A little consideration, tolerance and humor can go a
long way in allaying the fears of anxious parents. Even
complete failure with one family, despite a tremendous effort
should not offend or deflate the doctor's or student's ego.
Doctors' relationships with families sometimes don't gel; but
it is up to the doctor, who has the advantage, to recognize
this and to assist the parents and the small patient in
obtaining help elsewhere. This responsibility may lie with
some other doctor, an agency or other health professionals.
It may appear that the problem of only one patient is at
stake but usually the whole family is involved.

THE PEDIATRIC HISTORY

Over half of all diagnoses can be suspected, or even
made, from the history alone. The pediatric history often
involves a third party, namely the parent or guardian, and
depends on the age of the child. The toddler (1-4 years)
can be present when the history is taken from the parents
as this allows time for the child to learn that the doctor
is not a "terrifying person". Behavioral and emotional
problems and sordid environmental and family problems should
be discussed without the child. When the need so indicates,
utilize other relatives or the nurse as babysitters. The
details of organic symptoms should be checked with the

school aged child, but most of the history is best taken
with the child not present. With adolescents, two histories
should be taken separately - one from the child and one from
the parent. Each should have his day in court! Tactfully
excuse extraneous people who accompany the mother and child,
such as aunts, grandparents, neighbors, etc.

The parent may not recognize that certain changes are
significant and thus vital information may not be mentioned.
Accordingly, the history must be thorough, running down minor
leads to be sure they aren't major. Sometimes the key to
the problem may be revealed by the last question or remark
as the patient goes out of the door. A complete initial
history should be recorded and every organ system must be
checked on each occasion. Questions must be asked in terms
of how symptoms might appear from the mother's point of
view - e.g., ask about behavior that might suggest the child
is having headaches (or seizures) rather than ask if the
child has headaches (or seizures).

Verbal and facial clues may be missed if a checklist or
notebook is used. The informant should be faced and listened
to with minimal interruptions. The history must be told in
the parents' or the child's own words. If the mother states
that the infant is nervous and irritable, before sedating
the infant, make sure that it isn't the mother herself who
is overburdened by family problems.

Obtaining reliable information requires the full cooperation
and support of the informant (parent). Initially, the paren
must be permitted to talk freely about the problem or problems that concern her. Later a more direct or organized
history can be achieved. Since life styles differ, the interpretation of facts may not match the doctor's interpretation. Language should be geared to the parents' level of
understanding. This does not mean that the doctor should
talk down to the parent but rather that terms should be un-
derstandable. Contradiction should be avoided; a negative
reaction may inhibit or stop communication. Do not accept
acquiescence as evidence of understanding.

Always begin the history with whatever concerns the
parent the most. Hear these worries and complaints out with
little questioning but don't take more than notes at this
stage, for the real problem and the facts may not be in
proper sequence. To start, ask a general but friendly question, such as "Please tell me about Billy; what seems to
worry you?" or "How is Billy doing? Has he had any particular problems that concern you?"

Ascertain the nature, timing, duration, location, etc.
of symptoms and their response to treatment. Then go throug
the remainder of the history, noting and cross-referencing
any symptoms that might apply to the present illness (P.I.).
Don't hesitate to write the same fact twice.

ROLE OF PAST HISTORY

The genetic constitution, e.g. familial diseases -
require special care. Document precisely the relationships
to the child, not to the person giving the history. Check
for consanguinity, especially in cases of malformation or
inherited disease.

The mother's pregnancy must be checked: Her general
health? Any bleeding - if so, when? Excess vomiting?
Blood pressure and urine? Undue weight gain? Any infections
like rubella; if so, when? Any x-rays? Any drugs - vitamins?
iron? headache pills? nerve medicine? sleeping pills?
Labor - Was the baby born when expected - duration of labor?
Anesthesia? Head first? Forceps? Any complications? Neonatal -
Birth weight? General well being? Good cry? Sucked well?
Any blueness? Any jaundice? Needed O_2? What day did the
baby go home?

PHYSICAL EXAMINATION (POINTERS)

Make friends before starting the examination - play
with the child, examine a doll or animal. Talking and
smiling with an infant will often avert crying. Allow the
crying baby to suck on a pacifier or bottle. This frequently
will quiet him. Sometimes noticing the good looks or nice
dress of the child establishes good rapport. The toddler
should be examined in the mother's lap. If lying on a table
is frightening, the infant should be examined in the mother's

lap. Do as much as possible by inspection before approaching
the child. Warm hands and instruments as well as avoidance
of quick, rough movements produces better results. If the
child wishes to play with an instrument such as a stetho-
scope or ophthalmoscope, allow this. Be patient and relaxed
during the examination. If the doctor is tense and rushed,
the patient will tense up as well. If the child is old
enough to understand, explain what is going to be done and
demonstrate if possible. If the procedure is going to be
painful, be honest and say so without frightening the patient. The examination of the ears and throat bothers
infants and toddlers. Examine these last. For the older
toddler, it may be suitable to begin the examination with
eliciting the deep tendon reflexes. In the preschool child,
examination of the chest may be the best way to begin the
examination. In examining the abdomen, take time to put the
child at ease to achieve relaxation of the abdominal muscles.
Establish a methodological routine procedure for a physical
examination so as to avoid overlooking some areas. At times
the routine has to be changed, so don't be inflexible.

Remember to inspect first, then palpate and auscultate
or auscultate and palpate.

Most of all, enjoy the child and retain a sense of
humor. A little urine or regurgitant milk shouldn't be too
upsetting! Anticipate and take the necessary precautions.

STAGES OF DEVELOPMENT

1.   Intra Uterine

2.   Neonatal (Birth-4 weeks)

3.   Infancy (First 2 years)

4.   Pre-School period
     (2-6 years)

5.   Early school period
     6-10 years   Females
     6-12 years   Males

6.   Prepubescence
     10-12 years   Females
     12-14 years   Males

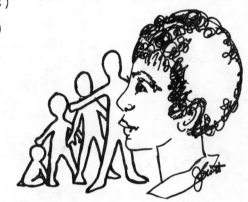

7.   Adolescence
     12-18 years   Females
     14-20 years   Males

These stages of development vary in different social classes. Life style, education, diet, and culture all affect this.[18] It has been shown that children in the USA mature physically 2 or 3 years earlier than children of the same age in parts of Europe.

SOCIAL AND ADAPTIVE DEVELOPMENT

Cultural attitudes and habits dictate the methods of handling and carrying infants. This affects motor activity, growth and psychological development of the infant.

Americans stroll infants in buggies; the English park babies in prams. Some people keep the baby all swaddled up. Some African mothers turn the newborn every two hours to avoid it lying in one position. Observe the baby and how it is handled. This will tell you a lot about the parents.

DEVELOPMENTAL MILESTONES
(SOCIAL AND ADAPTIVE)

4 WEEKS 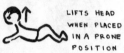 LIFTS HEAD WHEN PLACED IN A PRONE POSITION	**6-8 WEEKS** SMILES RESPONSIVELY	**3 MONTHS** BRINGS HANDS TOGETHER
4 MONTHS GRASPS OBJECTS 	**5 MONTHS** ROLLS OVER 	**6 MONTHS** REACHES FOR OBJECTS TRANSFERS RATTLE FROM HAND TO HAND
7 MONTHS SITS ALONE	**9-10 MONTHS** CRAWLS WAVES BYE-BYE	**11-12 MONTHS** PULLS UP TO A STANDING POSITION
12-14 MONTHS 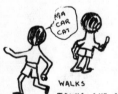 WALKS TALKS - ONE SYLLABLE WORDS.	**18 MONTHS** RUNS CLUMSILY UP STAIRS 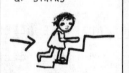	**20 MONTHS** CLIMBS DOWN STAIRS THROWS A BALL USES A SPOON NAMES ONE PICTURE
2 YEARS PEDALS BIKE VERBALIZES TOILET NEEDS	**3 YEARS** STATES AGE KNOWS SEX DRESSES WITH SUPERVISION	**4 YEARS** CATCHES BOUNCED BALL RECOGNISES 3 COLORS HOPS ON ONE FOOT

To thrive, babies need: Food
                           Comfort
                           Safety
                           Warmth
                           Stimulation

These variables affect the rate of learning and socialization, the conditioning and the response.[9]

WELL BABY VISITS

These visits can be used for parent education and to
pinpoint problems that are often easily handled.[10] Some
attention should be given to the mother to see if she is
having enough rest and if she is coping. A young mother may
have to stand up to parental criticism and intervention. In
multipara the baby may not be receiving enough attention.

The mother-child relationship can be assessed by noting
how the mother handles her baby.[17] Also observe the mother
while the baby is being examined to see if she is helping
or nonchalantly staring out of the window. A rough test of
the mother's attitude to the infant is to ask the mother what
she does if she has just fed the baby and changed the diaper
and he starts crying. If she says that she picks the baby
up, she scores 3; if she says she lets the baby cry, she
scores 0; and if she says that she rocks the baby, she scores
2. A low rating should cause one to check the mother. Remember, it is not enough just to think or believe that she
is an effective mother.

GROWTH AND DEVELOPMENT[14]

Psychological testing, measurements of height, length
and weight are repeated to ascertain the rate of growth of
the baby. In the first 6 months, if possible, these procedures should be performed monthly. In the last 6 months of
the year, they should be done twice. The better the nutritional and social level of a child, the earlier and more
rapid the onset of adolescence and the sooner growth is
completed.

When measuring, try to keep down the variables and be
consistent.

WEIGHT

Make sure that the scales are accurate. A wet diaper
one visit and a nude weight the next visit may reveal a
false weight loss and can be alarming. Always weigh the
baby in the nude.

During the first few days of the newborn period, some
weight loss occurs due to the passage of urine and meconium
and the low calorie intake. The weight loss is usually less
than 10% of the original birth weight and is regained by
the 7th to the 14th day. An assessment of weight gain during
the first year can be estimated as satisfactory if there is a
gain of 1/2 - 2 lbs. per month for the first 5 months (or 6-8
ounces per week), and 1 lb. per month from 5-12 months. Fat
babies may be overfed, but not well-nourished.

Approximate weights of infants and children (in lbs.):

Birth Weight	7.35 lbs.
3-12 months	age (mos.) + 11
1-6 years	age (yrs.) x 5 + 17
6-12 years	age (yrs.) x 7 + 5

A NORMAL INFANT USUALLY DOUBLES HIS BIRTH WEIGHT AT
5 MONTHS AND TRIPLES THE BIRTH WEIGHT AT ONE YEAR.

HEIGHT

Rates of growth vary. Check or note the size of parents
as shortness may be genetically determined. The average
body length at birth is 20 inches. At the end of the first
year it has increased by 50% and it has
doubled at the end of four years.

Measure from the same
end points. If you

measure on the right side, note that the right side was used
for length measurement. Start at the same spot. Measure
length from heel to head using the zero mark at the heel
base to the highest point on the occiput. See that the child
is lying as straight as possible. Always measure length and
head circumference while the child is flat on the back. Be
consistent and use the same units at each visit.

	Rule of Thumb
Birth	20"
1 year	30"
2-14 years	age (yrs.) x 2 1/2 + 30

PERCENTILE CHARTS

These charts are used to graph weight and height during
infancy. The percentile is based on comparing an infant or
child with 100 normal children. "Normals" can fall in the
range between the 3rd and 97th percentile. The shape of
the curve represents the rate of growth for an individual.
This is more important than the relative position of any
point on the curve, e.g. a child who follows the 10th percentile is much less worrisome than one who follows the 97th
percentile for a year and then drops to the 20th even though
the 20th is higher than the 10th percentile. A flattening
of the growth curve in the first year may suggest protein
deficiency. Remember that each child is an individual and
develops as such. It has been shown that differences in

the rate of growth also vary from one social class to another.

HEAD

Fontanelles (Soft Spots): There are two fontanelles, one
anterior and one posterior. Feel these and don't be afraid
to touch them. The anterior fontanelle may feel tense if
the baby is crying. In meningitis it may bulge. A depressed
anterior fontanelle suggests dehydration.

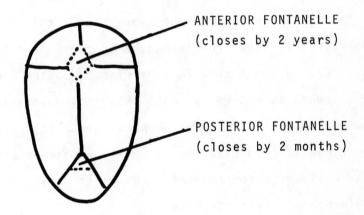

ANTERIOR FONTANELLE
(closes by 2 years)

POSTERIOR FONTANELLE
(closes by 2 months)

Circumference: Measure the head circumference to the nearest
half inch. Remember to measure using the same fixed points.
Head circumference at birth averages 13.5 inches ($\pm$ 1/2 inch).
This increases by 1/2 inch monthly for the first four months,
while a further two (2) inches are added in the remainder
of the first year. Watch for early fusion of the skull bones
(synostosis) or rapidly enlarging head size as seen in hydro-
cephalus.

	Age	Inches	Centimeters
	Birth	13.8	35.0
	3 mos.	15.9	40.4
	6 mos.	17.1	43.4
HEAD	9 mos.	17.8	45.3
	12 mos.	18.3	46.6
CIRCUMFERENCE	18 mos.	18.9	47.9
	2 yrs.	19.3	48.9
	2 1/2 yrs.	19.5	49.5
	3 yrs.	19.6	49.8
	5 yrs.	20.9	50.9

NEW BORN AND WELL BABY

In European countries such as Holland, the neonatal mortality is low and home delivery is the rule. Children are reared at home from day one. In other countries, newborns are put into sterile nurseries and often "rooming in", if allowed, is not encouraged. Hospital deliveries are routine in the USA and the neonatal mortality rate is one of the highest. Medical care may well need to be oriented to home deliveries for economic reasons as well as for lowering the neonatal mortality rate.

"Babies are born to live and not to die" and as such, the doctor's attitude should reflect one of optimism. Well babies provide the bulk of ambulatory pediatrics and therefore, a thorough knowledge of the normal is "a must" and will serve to alert to the abnormal.

APGAR SCORE

At birth, the newborn is exposed to a totally new environment and immediate adjustment is rated according to the "Apgar" score.

Apgar Score

	Sign	Score		
		0	1	2
A	Appearance	Blue; pale	Body pink	Completely pink
P	Pulse	Absent	Below 100	Over 100
G	Grimace (reflex irritability response to stimulation of sole of foot by glancing slap)	No response	Grimace	Cry
A	Activity	Limp	Some flexion of extremities	Active motion
R	Respiration	Absent	Slow; irregular	Good strong cry

This scoring system was devised to assist in the evaluation of the newborn and is assessed at one minute and 5 minutes after birth. Scores of 3 or below represent infants in very poor condition. The one minute score is a reflection of acid base status. The five minute score is a better reflection of oxygenation.

While in the nursery, the infant receives Silver Nitrate drops or penicillin ointment/drops in the eyes for protection against gonorrheal opthalmia. Sensitivity to penicillin can however develop. Vitamin K is administered to prevent hemorrhagic disease of the newborn. Before discharge home, a PKU test is done to detect phenylketonuria.

A NORMAL FULLTERM INFANT WEIGHS 2500 gms (5 1/2 lbs) OR MORE.

A lot of valuable information can be gained by looking at the newborn.[1] Note the general appearance of the newborn peaceful, sluggish or restless. Listen to the cry. The skin of the infant may be covered with extensive hair. This is known as LANUGO. A cheeselike white material VERNIX CASEOSA may be found in the creases and over the body (more pronounced in the premature infant). This coating does not need to be washed off since it evaporates.

Color: Look for jaundice (yellow discoloration) by examining the tip of the nose (when pressed and released). Jaundice on the first day or increasing jaundice may be due to excess red blood cell destruction and must be investigated and if necessary treated.

Cyanosis (generalized blue coloration): Must be dealt with promptly. To detect color changes, remember to examine the infant in natural light.

Muscle tone: Sedation during labor could cause the baby to be sluggish. Recheck if in doubt. Tone should be equal and firm.

Respiratory rate: This is normally 30-50 per minute. Respiratory distress may show itself as difficulty in sucking. Watch for fits or twitching. No stools or vomiting may indicate an obstruction, and pallor may suggest hemorrhage.

CHECK LIST

> MORE MISTAKES ARE MADE FROM NOT LOOKING THAN NOT KNOWING

UMBILICAL CORD: Examine for bleeding and infection. Make sure that there are two arteries and one vein.

CONGENITAL ABNORMALITIES: Look for spina bifida and imperforate anus. Examine the mouth and check for a cleft palate. A hare lip is frequently associated with a cleft palate.

CONGENITAL DISLOCATION OF THE HIP: Look at the buttocks creases - absence of the crease is suggestive of a dislocated hip. Feeling a click on abduction is diagnostic.

BIRTH INJURIES:

1. Cephalhematoma: This appears as rounded swelling on one side of the skull. It is due to subperiosteal hemorrhage and does not cross suture lines. No treatment is necessary. Reassure the mother that the swelling will disappear although it may take some weeks.

2. Caput Succudaneum: This is due to edema of the scalp and crosses suture lines. Involves the portion presenting during delivery.

3. Forceps Marks: May be associated with a facial nerve lesion due to pressure or damage and the infant may not move that side of the face. This usually improves on its own.

4.   Peripheral Nerve Injuries: May occur if there is
      injury to the brachial plexus. Erb-Duchenne para-
      lysis is limited to the 5th and 6th and Klumpke's
      is a rarer form of brachial plexus injury to the
      7th and 8th cervical nerves and the first thoracic.

MECONIUM: Check the diaper. All normal children should pass
a dark greenish-black meconium stool within the first 24
hours. If meconium is not passed in the first 24 hours the
baby must be observed and watched for intestinal obstruction.
By the third day, stools start to become normal in color.

HERNIAL ORIFICES: Examine inguinal region for hernias.
Umbilical hernias usually become evident at the toddler
stage.

THE HEART: Listen for murmurs. Check all pulses, especially
femorals, so you don't miss a coarctation of the aorta.

REFLEXES: There are many reflexes that can be looked for in
the newborn. Some examples are given below. Absence may be
due to the effect of drugs used on the mother during delivery
or may indicate the presence of neurologic abnormalities.

1.   Rooting reflex is obtained by touching the baby's
      cheek and noting the infant turn and suck. This
      is a normal reflex present at birth. Absence for
      more than 1 or 2 days is significant.

2.   Moro reflex occurs by startling the newborn. Star-
      tling is accomplished by making a loud noise:

bang on a table and observe the baby. Normally there is a reaction similar to grasping a tree. Absence denotes severe nervous system injury or deficiency. If the Moro persists after 5 months, it indicates definite pathology.

3.   Landau reflex occurs at 3 months. If you support the infant horizontally in a prone position, then the infant should a) raise his head, and b) arch his back.

THE PREMATURE INFANT

This is a high risk infant and is not uncommonly born to very young mothers, mothers who have toxemia of pregnancy, hypertension or diabetes or who have nutritional deficiencies such as protein deficiency or folic acid deficiency.[2]

A premature infant,[16] "preemie", is one born too early and therefore is not ready for independent life. Live born infants delivered before 37 weeks from the first day of the last menstrual period are considered to have a shortened gestational period and are termed premature. This definition is not as fixed as it sounds since only an estimate can be made of gestational dates and many infants although "early" for their dates are vigorous and well. Infants who weigh 2500 gms. or less (5 1/2 lbs.) are considered to have had either a shortened gestational period or a less than expected rate of intra-uterine growth, or both, and are classified as

low birth weight infants. Prematurity and low birth weight
usually occur together, particularly among infants weighing
1500 grams or less at birth and both are associated with
increased neonatal morbidity and mortality. In African hospitals a "preemie" may be an infant of under 4 1/2 lbs. in
weight as the incidence of prematurity is relatively high.
African infants weighing over 4 1/2 lbs. usually are not
given special care. American black babies at term weigh
500 gms. (average) less than white American babies. In
lower socioeconomic groups, women with multiple pregnancies
and/or poor nutrition who receive little or no prenatal medical care, the incidence of prematurity is high.

APPEARANCE

The appearance of the premature infant depends on how
much underweight the infant is. The premature baby will be
small, underweight, thin with a large head and abdomen. He
is also inactive with feeble movements and a poor cry. Respiration may be rapid and irregular. The sucking and swallowing reflex may be absent or feeble. The stomach is small
and "feeds" easily overflow and regurgitate into the lungs.
Body stores of vitamins and iron are far less than in a full
term infant. The premature infant's temperature varies
greatly as he cannot control it. The blood vessels are weak
walled and easily damaged. Severe jaundice can often occur
in the first few days of life. Developmental defects are

more common in the premature infant than in full term infants and often include impairment of intellectual or motor function.

The assessment of characteristics of the premature infant is dependent on experience and is often a matter of degree. The following table summarizes some characteristics of the premature infant.

Weight of Infant	1000 - 1500 grams	1500 - 2000 grams
Head size relative to body	Round and large	Less large
Skin and sub-cutaneous	Transparent appearance. No fat	More subcutaneous tissue
Tone	Atonic lie in tonic neck attitude little movement of extremities	Good when stimulated
Reflexes Moro Grasp	Weak Weak	Complete More vigorous
Cry	Weak	Strong cry
Sucking response	May be weak	Able to suck
Sleep pattern	Difficult to tell if asleep or awake	Easily discernible; able to fixate visually on some objects in their environment

The infant in the 2000 - 2500 gram category has the appearance of a small full term infant.

ASSESSMENT OF GESTATIONAL AGE AT BIRTH

Efforts have been made to differentiate the short gestation from the "small for the date" infant. Numerous reflexes, other signs and tests have been reported. A sense
of balance is needed. Physicians must first be able to
differentiate normal from abnormal and secondly detect neurological or biochemical defects that can be investigated
and treated. Knowing a host of reflexes without understandin
their significance doesn't help the infant or the parents.

A scoring system has been devised by Dubowitz[3] in order
to estimate the period of gestation. The external criteria
of Farr and associates[4] and the neurological criteria of
Dubowitz are rated. The lower the score, the more premature
the infant. The external characteristics measured are:
skin color, skin texture, skin opacity, edema, lanugo, ear
form, ear firmness, genitals, breast size, nipple formation,
and plantar skin creases.

Plantar Skin Creases: Until 36 weeks of gestation there are
only one or two transverse skin creases on the sole of the
foot anteriorly. By 37 or 38 weeks more creases have appeare
and by 40 weeks there is a complete series of crisscrossed
creases covering the entire sole.

Size of the Breast Nodule: This correlates generally with
gestational age. It is usually not palpable at 33 weeks.
At 36 weeks it is under 3 mm. in diameter and in term infants

it is usually 4-10 mm.

Scalp Hair: Up to 37 weeks it is short and fuzzy. At 40
weeks it consists of silky strands.

Ear Lobe Cartilage: Cartilage of the ear lobe, which makes
the folds of the helix and antihelix stand out, develops
chiefly between 36 and 40 weeks.

Genitalia: At 36 weeks the testes have not descended completely and the Scrotal Rugae are limited to the anterior
and inferior aspects of the scrotum. By 40 weeks the testes
are usually descended and rugae cover the entire scrotal
surface. In the female by 40 weeks (with the legs half
abducted) labia majora cover the labia minora.

FEEDING PROBLEMS

The premature infant requires more calories/lb. to gain
weight than the full term infant, e.g. 60 + calories per lb.
or 120 + calories per kilo. The average premature infant
gains 6-7 kg. (13-15 lbs.) in the first year. These infants
have less resistance during the first year of life and must
be protected from infections. In addition, the premature
infant requires added iron in the diet because iron stores
are built up in the body during the last two months of gestation. (15 mgs. of reduced iron is given per day).

The premature infant is more difficult to nurse. He
may require smaller feeds, get cold easier and have a more
anxious mother, especially if the baby and mother have been

separated for some time and the mother has been allowed
minimal handling of the infant. Allowing the mother to be
a participant during the time of careful nursing can make
her more confident.

INFANT FEEDING

Some women have strict regimes or schedules and feed
the infant with clock work regularity at four hour intervals
only, with measured amounts of milk. This regularity is
easier when bottle feeding but should be avoided if possible.
Demand feeding is by far the better approach. The newborn
cries, eats, feeds, sleeps and may require 8 to 10 feeds a
day until a more regular rhythm is established at approximately 2 months. About this time, the infant often starts
looking around at the surroundings and feeds less - about
5 or 6 times a day. Demand feeding can be overdone and the
mother should be reassured that every time the baby cries,
food is not the need. The baby should be checked for a wet
diaper, an opened diaper pin, or should be dewinded. A
mother gets to know the different cries of the baby. A
little cuddling, cooing and warmth often quiet the baby.
BREAST OR BOTTLE?

Methods of infant feeding must be varied for families
of different social and educational standards. The individual preferences of mothers are important deciding factors
as to whether breast feeding or artificial feeding is used.

Women of lower economic groups, those in under-developed
countries without refrigeration or running water, or the
poor who can't afford to buy artificial food have no choice
but to breast feed. Professional women tend to prefer
breast feeding. In the USA 80-90% of newborn infants are
artificially fed in contrast to African babies 80-90% of
whom are breast fed. Some pediatricians tend to favor bottle
feeding because they know more about artificial than natural
feeding.

The ideal food for babies is breast milk and it provides
essential nutrients and calories.

	Protein	Fat	Sugar
Breast Milk	1.5%	4%	7%
Cow's Milk	5%	4-5%	4-5%

The composition of milk varies and the above are approximate percentages. The essential fatty-acid content of
human milk is three times greater than that of cow's milk.

The number of calories that milk provides varies according to the type of milk:

One Ounce	Provides
Breast Milk	20 calories
Cow's Milk	20 calories
Evaporated Milk	40 calories
Karo & Sugar (carbohydrate)	120 calories

The caloric requirement for full term infants during
the first six months is 50-55 calories per pound of body
weight per twenty-four hours. This gradually decreases to
45 calories per pound. While breast feeding is the ideal
or preferred infant feed, the choice of type of feeding is
the mother's. If she prefers bottle feeding, do not make
her feel guilty. Some women find nursing unsatisfactory.
Basic psychologic feelings interfere with the success of
breast feeding. If on the other hand she wishes to breast
feed, encourage her to do so.

BREAST FEEDING[8]

The onset of the production of breast milk starts about
the third day after delivery. Colostrum precedes the secretion of milk and this is high in antibodies, protein and
minerals (zinc and iron). It is low in fat and carbohydrate
content.

THE MOTHER WHO BREAST FEEDS MUST HAVE AN ADEQUATE DIET
containing twice as many calories as she would normally eat
and at least 3 quarts of fluid per day. She should eat a
balanced diet, get rest and exercise to improve muscle tone.

Reassure the mother that breast feeding does not harm
the breast contour. If the mother finds feeding too con-
fining, a supplemental cow's milk bottle can be given occasionally to free the mother for a few hours. Remind the
mother who is nursing not to use suppositories or any drugs
unless she has checked with her doctor.

Some babies receive enough milk from one breast. Others need to nurse at both breasts. At each feeding one breast needs to be emptied because emptying the breast is the best galactogogue. While feeding the mother should assume a comfortable position. Most of all, she should relax and enjoy feeding her baby. Feeding can last from 10 minutes to 30 minutes. Most babies average 20-30 minutes at the breast, but there is no time limit to breast feeding. If there has been a long interval between feeds, check to see that the breasts are not engorged. Sometimes the mother may have to express the breast so there is a good steady flow. Breast fed babies have looser stools than bottle fed babies, but sometimes several days may go by with no stool being passed. This is normal with a breast fed baby. Solids may be added to the diet of the breast fed baby on the same schedule as they are fed to the artificially fed baby. Care of the nipples should not become a ritual. The mother can easily clean her breasts with water while bathing, but should avoid soaping them.

The Advantages of Breast Feeding

1.   Breast milk has an ideal composition for babies.

2.   Nursing stimulates involution of the uterus after delivery.

3.   Babies are far less prone to infections during the first year of life.

4. Milk allergies do not occur in breast fed babies.

5. Atopic eczema is seven times more common in the artificially fed baby.

6. There is great psychological satisfaction for both the mother and the infant. It promotes a togetherness.

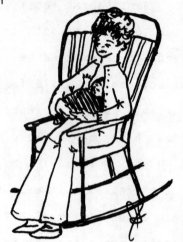

7. The method is easy and convenient.

8. The incidence of breast cancer is lower in nursing mothers.

FORMULA FEEDING OR ARTIFICIAL FEEDS

If the mother does not wish to breast feed, then instruct her carefully as to the:

1. Type of milk preparation to use.

2. How to prepare it correctly.

3. The quantity to give per feed.

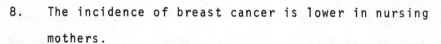

Give the mother written instructions as well as verbal. Diagrams may be useful. Remember to stress the importance of cuddling the baby and talking to the baby. Warn against the bottle propping technique that deprives the baby of love and tenderness.

There are many prepared formulas on the market today, most of which are prepared to resemble breast milk. Some are already prepared for feeding (instant type) and others must be diluted with an equal amount of water. Whether the milk is diluted or not each ounce is so prepared that it provides 20 calories. These preparations can be very expensive. The least expensive formula is an evaporated milk with Karo syrup or cane sugar added, or diluted cow's milk with sugar or Karo added.

Preparation: Small infants are not given high protein diets because their kidneys are unable to excrete the end products of protein metabolism in large amounts. Milk is high in protein, so carbohydrate and water is always added to milk to make a formula.

COW'S MILK FORMULA

Milk	2 parts
Water	1 part
Carbohydrate	1 ounce

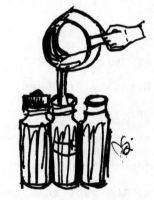

EVAPORATED MILK FORMULA

Evaporated Milk	1 part
Water	2 parts
Cane sugar or Karo syrup	1 ounce = 2 Tbsps.

The calculation of calories provided for a 10 lb. infant on evaporated milk formula would be:

```
Evaporated milk      10 ounces      10 x 40 = 400
Water                20 ounces
Karo syrup           1 ounce        1 x 120 = 120
                                    calories:  520
```

The daily intake would be 50 calories per lb.

Depending on the infant's weight the quantities required vary as follows:

Weight	EM[+](oz)	+Water (oz)	+Karo (Tbsps)	=Calories
6 lbs.	6	12	2	360
7 lbs.	7	14	2	400
8 lbs.	8	16	2	440
9 lbs.	9	18	2	480
10 lbs.	10	20	2	520
11 lbs.*	13	19	2	640

*11 lbs. and over combination provides 32 ounces (1 quart) per day and this is the upper limit
[+]EM = Evaporated Milk

For babies with milk allergy, hypo allergic milk such as soya milk meat base preparations or Nutramigen work well. Quantity Per Feed: The newborn may take 1 1/2 to 2 ounces per feed, gradually increasing the amount per feed. After the first few months the frequent feeds are reduced to 3-4 feeds per day by the time the infant is 6 months old, due to the fact that the emptying time of the stomach becomes less frequent.

Infants vary as to the number of feeds they need and the quantity of formula at each feeding. Some infants require milk every 3 hours, some every four hours and still others at longer intervals.

SOLIDS (WEANING)

In the USA solids are introduced early. Be careful that the mother doesn't overfeed the baby with starches when solids are introduced. SOLIDS ARE INTRO-DUCED AT ABOUT SIX WEEKS OF AGE, usually when the infant returns for the first newborn visit. The most important aspect is that each new food be given separately so that if there is an allergy to any food it can be detected easily. The infant is usually started on cereals (which are prepared and milk added), then fruits are added and later vegetables. Remember: Solids should be fed from a spoon and not in the bottle. At first the infant will attempt to suck from the spoon, so place the spoon in the middle of the tongue to avoid the expulsion of the food from the mouth. The mother should not be discouraged if the infant seems to reject spoon feeding. Do not make a major issue of it, just dis-continue and try another time. It often helps to try another food, e.g. banana is readily accepted, prunes may not be. Note which foods were rejected as well as those accepted.

Baby foods: used initially, are pureed

Junior foods: chopped and given at 6-7 months of age

Table foods: mashed and given at 6-7 months of age

Babies can be overfed and evidence would suggest that obesit
later in life may be related to overfeeding in infancy,
especially when using artificial feeds and early solids.

Vitamins and Iron

Vitamins A, D, and C should be supplemented starting
about 2-4 weeks after birth and continued during the baby's
first year. Fluoride should also be added if there is no
fluoridation of water in a city. 15 mgs. of reduced iron is
given prophylactically as Fer-in-sol 0.6 ccs. daily for the
first 6-9 months until the child goes onto table food. However, it has been shown that excess iron intake may interfere with copper metabolism and cause hemolytic anemia.

IMMUNIZATIONS[12,15]

This is an important part of well baby care. Make sure
that you chart any immunizations given and also that you
tell the mother what is being given and let her keep her own
record.

Immunizations are not to be given in the presence of
fever or of illness. Interruption of routine immunization
schedule because of illness, failure to keep appointments,
etc. causing a delay between doses will not interfere with
the final immunity and the series of shots need not be
started again, regardless of the interval between immunizations.

VACCINATION

Recently, smallpox vaccination was discontinued in the USA as a routine immunization since more children died from vaccination than from smallpox. However, in countries where smallpox has not been erradicated, compulsory vaccination is required in the first year.

IMMUNIZATION SCHEDULE[15]

Age	Immunizing Agent
2 months	DPT #1 + OPV Trivalent
4 months	DPT #2 + OPV Trivalent
6 months	DPT #3 + OPV Trivalent
12 months	Tuberculin Test Rubeola + Rubella combined or measles-mumps-rubella combined vaccines
18 months	DPT + OPV Trivalent Booster
3 years	Tuberculin Test
4-6 years	DPT + OPV Trivalent; Tuberculin Test
1-12 years	Mumps if not given with measles-rubella
14-16 years	DT (Adult) DT (Adult) q. 10 years thereafter

OPV - ORAL POLIO VACCINE (3 shots)

1. Oral vaccine should not be given at less than 6 week intervals.

2. Infants under 1 year of age who have received Monovalent series should receive the Trivalent booster 1 year later and before entering school. In pre-school children, the booster may be omitted.

3.   Infants and pre-school children first receiving Triva-
      lent vaccine after 6 months of age require 2 doses, 8
      weeks apart plus a booster in 1 year and one before
      entering school.

DPT - DIPHTHERIA, PERTUSSIS AND TETANUS SHOTS (3 shots)

      Start only after 4 weeks of age and give at a minimum
of 4 week intervals. If a child has a severe reaction to a
DPT injection (e.g. high fever or convulsion usually due to
the pertussis vaccine) either give only D or T omitting the
pertussis vaccine. Desensitize the infant with very small
injections of the pertussis vaccine. Always ask the mother
to inform you if there is a reaction before continuing the
immunization.

TUBERCULIN TESTING

      This is usually done at the end of the first year unless
there has been exposure to the disease or the infant has an
illness which may be tuberculosis. The test should be repeated every 18-24 months. In high risk populations or
where there is individual exposure, checking may need to be
more frequent. Remember to check the family members and
contacts. The tuberculin test must be performed before the
rubeola vaccine is given or at least 2 months after the
rubeola vaccine, for this vaccine suppresses a positive test

      Infants and children who are likely to be exposed to
adults with recently arrested pulmonary or renal tuberculosis

may be given INH but the indications must be clear-cut because
there are side effects. In children with active tuberculosis
or a positive tuberculin test, treatment must be started
before rubeola vaccine is given.

MEASLES VACCINE

Two types of attenuated live measles are available:
1) Edmonston B vaccine with or without immune serum globulin
and 2) Attenuated vaccines (Schwartz and Moraten). Using
either vaccine, 30% of children develop a reaction consisting
of a high fever 103° F. or more for 2-5 days commencing on
the 6th day after injection. A modified rash may develop
in 40% of patients when the fever subsides. A few children
develop a mild cough and coryza. Contraindications to live
measles vaccine are pregnancy, leukemia, lymphoma or other
malignancies, therapy which depresses resistance and immunity
such as steroid treatment, irradiation antimetabolites, al-
kylating agents and untreated tuberculosis.

COMMON CONDITIONS

UMBILICAL HERNIA

This is a protrusion of the umbilicus. It is more
common in blacks. The majority of umbilical hernias disappear by 2 years of age, when walking is well established.
Tapes, etc. do not hasten the closure. They only serve to
hide the hernia and adhesives often cause irritation of the

skin. There is no danger regardless of the size; it is just
cosmetically unattractive.

RASHES

Rashes are very common and usually are due to local ski
irritants, e.g. soaps, oils, lotions. Occasionally an infan
develops a rash due to a food allergy, so ask about the type
of feeding and when new foods were introduced. Foods commonly causing rashes: wheat, chocolate, eggs, fish, milk
and citrus fruits.

Diaper rash is due to the detergents used on diapers
and often occurs in diapers which are perfumed. Common aggra
vation is rubber or plastic pants which prevent evaporation
of urine. Sensitivity to "Pampers" may be the cause of the
rash.

MONILIASIS (Thrush)

If the child has moniliasis of the mouth, check the
buttocks, genitalia and also look behind the ears for weepin
lesions. Make sure that the mother has not got vaginal moniliasis because she will also need to be treated.

DIARRHEA

Normally a breast fed baby may have 3 to 5 fairly thin
bright yellow stools. The artificially fed baby usually has
fewer stools. They are lighter in color and more formed.
When a baby has diarrhea, the stools are watery, may be yellow or green in color, contain mucus and are foul smelling.

To treat diarrhea, the baby is usually put on clear fluids until stooling stops and then gradually diluted milk and other foods are added to the diet.

CONSTIPATION

What the mother means by "constipation" must be clarified. All infants do not have a stool each day. If the stool is hard and difficult to pass, then fruit juices or stool softeners may have to be used. Do not administer laxatives or soap inserted into the rectum. Inspect for anal fissure (small tear around anus). Straining is not necessarily due to constipation and the stool may be soft. Remember, in breast fed babies stools may be absent for several days.

COLIC

Excessive crying the first few months, not relieved by anything and disappearing after 6-12 weeks, has been attributed to colic. Make sure that all other causes are ruled out.

CRYING

Remember that the baby's contact with the environment is via the oral route and a cry may denote pain, boredom, or hunger, and is best interpreted by the mother.

SNEEZING

This is normal in the newborn and usually indicates infant's cleaning of the nasal cavity.

ACCIDENTS

Accidents are the most common cause of death during the first years of a child's life. Such accidents include falls burns, inhalation of foreign objects, poisoning, e.g. lead from eating chipped paint, soil, burning of batteries for fuel, etc.; aspirin poisoning is extremely common and rat poison is occasionally eaten (because it looks like peanut butter). Children like to put different things into their mouths. Pica eating is most common in the 1-3 year old grou All of these accidents are preventable and the mother should be instructed as to what simple precautions to take. It should not be assumed that the mother knows that dangerous chemicals, household aids, pesticides and medicines should be kept in locked cupboards. The parents should be specifically warned about accident prevention as most accidents do occur in the house.

ACUTE CONDITIONS

If any of the following complaints are cited by the mother, have her bring the baby into the office or clinic. Any of these conditions requires immediate investigation.

1.   Fever
2.   Vomiting
3.   Suddenly not taking the breast or the bottle (may suggest difficulty in breathing or anorexia)
4.   Apnoea
5.   Cyanosis

6. Rashes
7. Twitching and convulsions
8. Bloody stools or stools with mucus
9. Sudden weight loss

Educate the parents about the main conditions needing immediate attention. Nurse practitioners and pediatric assistants are now providing valuable continuity care, well child care, counseling and screening. Hopefully this will allow pediatricians more time with sick children and their parents.

REFERENCES

1. Barness L: Manual of Pediatric Physical Diagnosis.
    Chicago, Year Book Medical Publishers, 1969

2. Baumslag N, Edelstein T, Metz J: Reduction of inci-
    dence of prematurity by folic acid supplementation in
    pregnancy. BMJ 1:16, 1970

3. Dubowitz L, Dubowitz V, Goldberg C: Clinical assessment
    of gestational age in the newborn infant. J Ped 77:1,
    1970

4. Farr V, Kerridge DF, Mitchell RG: The value of some
    external characteristics in the assessment of gesta-
    tional age. Devel Med Child 8:657, 1966

5. Green M, Haggerty RF: Ambulatory Pediatrics. Phila-
    delphia, W.B. Saunders, 1968

6. Heaggerty MC: The use of the telephone in pediatric
    practice. Ambulatory Pediatrics. Edited by M Green,
    RJ Haggerty. Philadelphia, W.B. Saunders, 1968

7. Incest and the family disorder. BMJ 2:364, 1972
    (Editorial)

8. Jelliffe DB, Jelliffe EFP: The uniqueness of human
    milk. Amer Jour of Clinical Nutrition 24:970, 1971
    (Symposium)

9. Konner MJ: Newborn walking: Additional data. Science
    179:307, 1973

10. Leavitt R, Gofman H, Harvin D: Use of developmental
    charts in teaching well child care. Pediatrics 31:
    499, 1963

11. Mattson A: Long-term physical illness in childhood:
    A challenge to psychosocial adaptation. Pediatrics
    50:801, 1972

12. Morbidity and Mortality. Volume 21, Number 25, 1972.
    Supplement Collected Recommendations of the Public
    Health Service Advisory Committee on Immunization
    Practices

13. Nelson MM, Forfar JO: Associations between drugs ad-
    ministered during pregnancy and congenital abnormalities
    of the fetus. BMJ 1: 523, 1971

14.   Nelson V, McKay: Textbook of Pediatrics.   Philadelphia,
      W.B. Saunders, 1968

15.   Report of the Committee on Infectious Diseases.   Illinois,
      American Academy of Pediatrics, 1971

16.   Robinson R: The preterm baby.   BMJ 4:416, 1971

17.   Stone FH: Psychological aspects of early mother-infant
      relationship.   BMJ 4:224, 1971

18.   Williams DC, Jelliffe DB: Mother and Child Health:
      Delivering the Services.   New York, Oxford University
      Press, 1972

BOOKS FOR PARENTS

1.   Dittman L: The Mentally Retarded Child at Home.
     Washington, U.S. Dept H.E.W., Children's Bureau Publi-
     cation No. 374, 1959

2.   Newton N: The Family Book of Child Care.   New York,
     Harper, 1957

3.   Pryor K: Nursing Your Baby.   New York, Harper and Row,
     1963

4.   Spock B: Baby and Child Care.   New York, Hawthorne,
     1970

The Abnormal Child

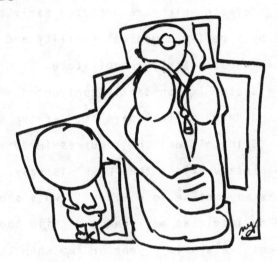

THE MAJORITY OF infants are born healthy. One in
    forty however have malformations, deformities or
seases which will seriously impair health, adversely affect
velopment and disturb the function of the family.[6,7]

Many of these babies benefit by being brought up in
eir natural homes.[1] For parents to accept their handi-
pped child at home however, they must want to do so. If
ey do not want to do so, the child must be institutionalized
d this may be economically crippling to the family, and
en detrimental to the child. Ironically, some of the

123

institutions that have been set up to help the severely handicapped are often totally ineffective. There are however
medical and social services available that can alleviate a
lot of unnecessary difficulty. For instance, visual and
auditory defects which are detected early can be successfully
handled by a well-run medical facility and the handicapped
child can be adequately rehabilitated.

The doctor is constantly confronted with the problem of
"when" and "how" to tell parents. If the abnormality is
obvious (Spina bifida) and requires immediate medical or
surgical intervention, the "when" is easy. However, the
diagnosis may not be so obvious (Down's syndrome or mongolism
and the pediatrician may send the child home only to have
the parents return in a year or two when the clinical manifestations present. If there is doubt, carefully communicate
it to the parents so that the child can be monitored during
his development. If the parents are going to have the respon
sibility of caring for the child, all the medical knowledge
should be made available to them.

The doctor who has had the most contact with the family
should be the one to tell the parents. He should state the
problem, discuss the doubts in diagnosis if there are any,
indicate the types of tests needed and if possible give them
some idea of how long these tests are going to take. Parents
should be given an opportunity to ask questions and also be

encouraged to do so. Each case must be treated on an individual basis since parents react differently. General guidelines for the parents should be offered. They should be
told about clinical manifestations and how to handle them in
all situations. Reassure them that there is no social dis-
grace associated with a handicapped child. They should be
advised how and what to inform other members of the family.
This is particularly important for the siblings who will have
to deal with the questions and remarks of school friends.
Parents will also have to learn to define limits for the
child. Permissiveness, recriminations and neglect should be
guarded against. The main object is for the doctor to "see"
the abnormal child in the home setting and anticipate the
problems the family will have to handle.

Subsequent meetings should be arranged with the primary
physician, the consultant where necessary, and other competent sympathetic personnel who will offer practical advice
and provide continuity of care on an outpatient or home visit
basis.[3] Information regarding special agencies, means of
obtaining appliances, transportation, special camps, financial aid or other specific resources should be given. Information about parent groups also may be helpful. Try to
anticipate the family needs and actively provide assistance.

When death occurs in the newborn, it is attended by
variable degrees of grief.[2,5,8] It has been found to be

more marked in mothers who have not had time or the opportunity to discuss it with their husbands. The reaction is
also more severe where there has been a previous stillbirth
or where the mother has had a chance to handle the baby.[4]
Feelings of guilt or inadequacy may result, and several
meetings may have to be arranged with the parents in order
to help them handle their feelings and realistically come to
terms with the situation.

REFERENCES

1. Adams M: Social aspects of medical care for the mentally retarded. New Eng J Med 286:635, 1972

2. Early deaths. BMJ 4:315, 1971   (Editorial)

3. Hide DW, Semple C: Coordinated care of the child with Spina bifida. Lancet 2:603, 1970

4. Kennel JH, Slyter H, Klaus MH: The mourning response of parents to the death of a newborn infant. New Eng J Med 283:344, 1970

5. Kozol J: Death at an Early Age. New York, Bantam, 1970

6. Mattson: Long-term physical illness in childhood: A challenge to psycho-social adaptation. Pediatrics 50: 801, 1972

7. National Association for Mental Health Working Party: Birth of an abnormal child: Telling the parents. Lancet 2:1075, 1971

8. Sudden deaths in infants. Lancet 2:1070, 1971 (Editorial)

CHAPTER 5

Child Abuse

ROBERT M. REECE

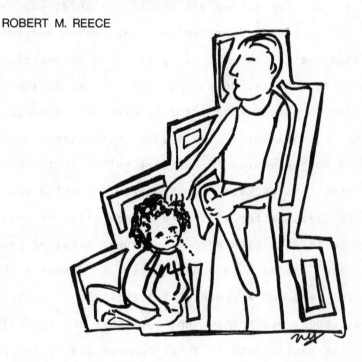

RATIONALIZATIONS HAVE BEEN made for the violence
which is so prominent in every aspect of our daily
lives. Crowding and traffic problems, pollution of streams,
lakes and air by industrial and automobile emissions, as
well as pollution of the mind by poorly motivated radio,
television and movies are all part of our culture. Lethal
weapons of every type and realistic war games and toy guns
are bought and sold over and under the counter to all age

groups.   Drugs are peddled and pushed and pills are available for the slightest symptom of pain or strain.

In this setting children in many rural areas and in most of our core cities are badly nourished, poorly tolerated for their youthful shortcomings, and denied adequate health care and health counseling. Increasing financial burdens and constant social demands tend to put an unreasonable pressure on parents who react by blaming and consequently alienating the youth. The traditional concept that the married mother and/or the natural mother is the best mother completes this backdrop for the drama of child abuse.

In 1946, Caffey's[1] initial description of multiple fractures in infants with chronic subdural hematoma prompted Silverman[14] to postulate and Kempe[11] to document that such injuries were not accidental but inflicted. Child abuse is not a sudden, new phenomenon, but there are indications that it is increasing both in total numbers and in the percentage of children involved.[5,15] The Society for the Prevention of Cruelty to Animals antedated by several decades the Society for the Prevention of Cruelty to Children and by many more years, the formation of the Childrens' Protective Service, an agency primarily concerned with counseling of parents. Perhaps this reflects the reluctance of society to examine or interfere with traditional parental control of the family unit in decisions of childrearing.   For the less blatant

forms of child abuse have often masqueraded as acceptable
disciplinary practices, and those critical of standard practices are considered invaders of privacy.

The battered child has been defined as "any child who
received non-accidental physical injury (or injuries) as a
result of acts (or omissions) on part of his parents or
guardians".[8,12] Other forms of child care lapses are poor
environmental control[6] and repetitive accidental poisonings.[3]
Sexual abuse is probably differently motivated and therefore
is not considered part of the syndrome. No age limits are
described, but in most situations, abuse refers to the pre-
pubertal child.

INCIDENCE

A national survey of reported cases during 1967 and
1968 revealed a total of seven thousand cases, but this represented only episodes reported through legal channels.[5]
Although all states have reporting laws, they are not uni-
form. The true incidence also remains elusive because
abusing parents have a wide spectrum of available medical
contacts especially in urban areas allowing them to maintain
the aura of "new patients" to successive health teams which
they often seek out only after the trauma has significantly
subsided. In 1970, New York City had over 2,700 cases reported. Kempe and Helfer feel that a reasonable accurate
estimate based on figures derived from their studies in

Denver, is 250-300 cases reported per million population per year.[12] If this figure is accurate, extrapolation would give national figures of over 50,000 battered children annually. The case fatality rates in the 1960's, also derived from reported cases only, comprised in most studies eleven to twenty-seven percent of cases. Permanent brain damage in survivors ranged from eight to thirty-one percent. However, these figures may not be truly reliable and new epidemiologic and followup data are needed.

CLINICAL MANIFESTATIONS

PSYCHOLOGICAL SIGNS AND SYMPTOMS

Extreme fright, whimpering, attempts to hide under the sheets, or profound apathy, stupor, and blunting of affect are the two most characteristic modes of the battered child syndrome. The patient may lie motionless, devoid of all facial expression. There is usually no bizarre behavior and consequently it is not difficult to distinguish him from the schizophrenic or autistic child. One gets the feeling that his "inner psychic life has been suspended".[4]

These patterns change during hospitalization. The child's affect progresses from initial passivity through fright to increasingly active behavior. He begins to eat and his appetite for human contact becomes so strong that he becomes clinging. This is the child who is often seen in the arms of a nurse of House Officer on rounds in the hospital. The socialization process in the child undergoes a rapid acceleration and consequently, at the time of his discharge, he may evidence a gain of as much as six months maturity in the areas of social, psychologic/intellectual and motor development.

PHYSICAL SIGNS

Usually there is evidence of numerous traumatic episodes and a discrepancy may exist between the findings and the historical account of the "accident". Significantly, no new lesions appear during hospitalization, distinguishing the maltreatment syndrome from other initial diagnostic considerations. The external injuries may include cuts, abrasions, burns, fractures, soft tissue injuries, and hematomata. Examine the fundi for retinal hemorrhage, detached retina or traumatic cataracts. Examine the mouth for missing or fractured teeth plus tears in the mucus membranes. The frenulum of the upper lip may be repeatedly traumatized by blows on the mouth. Ruptured or hemorrhagic ear drums suggests blows on the ears. Sometimes there is an inability to move limbs, head and neck. There can be neurological signs of brain damage. Convulsions, coma or death may constitute the extreme neurological insult. Exaggerated startle reflex, hyper-reflexia and increased muscle tone, however, are sometimes the only positive neurological findings, if indeed, any are present.

RADIOGRAPHIC SIGNS

Gross new and old fractures are present. Skeletal injuries have a predilection for the epiphyses and metaphyses. There are exaggerated periosteal reactions and a multiplicity of lesions in differing stages of healing is present. Since the periosteum is loosely attached in infants, it is easily separated and sub-periosteal hemorrhage is common. Calcium is deposited on the under surface of the periosteum within two to three weeks. New bone formation proceeds and long bones are remodeled by the healing process. Soft tissue injuries are evidenced by swelling and obliteration of muscular septa. Intra-abdominal injury may be manifested by pneumo-peritoneum, hemoperitoneum or ileus.

Despite the fact that injuries to some children are very severe, most injuries do not require hospitalization. Hospitalization may be advisable, however, to provide temporary separation from the caretakers, thus affording time to investigate and depressurize the social and psychological forces operating in the family constellation.

DIFFERENTIAL DIAGNOSIS

Few conditions are confused with the battered child if adequate historical, psychological and social assessments are made. The following disease states have certain similarities and differences. The differential points are listed below:

SYPHILIS

In this disease, bone lesions are symmetrical, other stigmata of syphilis (skin lesions, deformed teeth, paralyses) may be present, and a positive serology is usually present.

SCURVY

The bones have a ground glass appearance on x-ray with generalized demineralization, the vitamin C level of the serum is low, and epiphyseal ringing (Wimberger's ring) is often present on the radiograph.

OSTEOGENESIS IMPERFECTA

This condition is seen during the first three months of life and almost always involves the mandible (95%), clavicles, scapula and ribs.

OSTEOID OSTEOMA

Osteoma has no metaphyseal lesions and a nidus at the center of the lesion is diagnostic.

COAGULAPATHIES

Diseases of coagulation may be ruled out by appropriate clotting studies and platelet assessment.

THE FAMILY OF THE BATTERED CHILD

The parents of an abused child have been variously described as immature, rigid, impulsive, compulsive, self-centered, hypersensitive, quick to react, sociopathic, alcoholic and/or sexually promiscuous persons, often exhibiting poorly controlled aggression. Not uncommonly, investigation

of a parent's background reveals that he or she has also
been a battered child.

The maltreated child is often conceived premaritally
and unwanted (over fifty percent of the cases in one study).
This child may be either the single victim in the family or
just the one with a visible defect such as harelip, phoco-
melia, orthopedic or dermatologic abnormalities, or simply
one of low birth weight.[10]

A battered child is frequently made a symbol of parental
hostility to society. The parents may speak of him as if
he were already an adult with all of the adult's capacity
for deliberate, purposeful and organized behavior.[4] While
most parents consider a child's traits as tentative or potential indicators of adult qualities, the abusive parent may
see the child as currently possessing these qualities.

Inexperienced health workers and lay people often consider the abusive parent to be psychotic, but Helfer and
Kempe[12] assert that most professionals working in this field
feel that less than 10% of abusing parents are psychotic.
Most of the maltreated children can be returned to their
homes within one year of the reported abuse, given a sound
therapeutic program. Moreover, Helfer and Kempe, on the
basis of extensive surveys, have developed a patient profile
to predict potential abusive parents. The profile consists
of four major socio-psychologic parameters:

1.   Assessment of the quality of the parent's own up-
bringing to determine the degree of mothering received.

2.   Assessment of the parent's involvement with his
family and the community in which he lives.

3.   Assessment of the spouse's ability to support,
give love and maintain activity in the family relationships.

4.   Assessment of the presence and the degree of unrealistic expectations for the child by the parents.

When a parent who has inadequacies in the above cate-
gories, has a child who is either actually different (physical or emotional abnormalities), or is perceived as different
by the parent and a major or minor crisis is introduced into
the environment, it is very likely that the child will suffer
some form of abuse.

THE ROLE OF PROFESSIONALS

Who are the progessionals involved in a child abuse
problem? There are few fields in medicine where a more
multifaceted approach is required. Physicians (primary,
surgical, psychiatric), nurses, social workers (intake and
agency), policemen, legal authorities, psychologists, news
media personnel, hospital administrators, and emergency
medical transport operators are all involved in the process.

INTERVENTION

A system for recognition of the problem and initiation
of appropriate and parentally acceptable intervention requires

coordinated planning. At present, the usual first medical
contact in child abuse is the emergency room physician. In
smaller communities or in non-training hospitals this physician may be a full-time employee of the emergency room or
in private practice fulfilling rotation for the hospital.
In larger cities where residency programs are common, it
is likely that the first contact is a young physician in the
early stages of training, inexperienced in complex socio-
psychological medical cases. While directors of training
programs should endeavor to heighten the physician's level
of suspicion of possible abuse, it is essential that the new
physician learn specifically to avoid premature confrontation
or explication of the problem to abusing parents. Natural
anger and indignation should be suppressed and a non-punitive
and non-judgmental approach must be adopted.

The hospital has a particular set of obligations to
fulfill through the combined efforts of administration, socia
and psychiatric services, and the medical staff, a fully
understood and literal procedure should be formulated and
implemented. This should instruct all levels of personnel
regarding the issues and policies which pertain to cases of
suspected child abuse. Legal counsel is helpful to apprise
the hospital of local laws concerning child abuse.

The inter-relationships of the medical, nursing and
social service staffs, with periodic case conferences

involving all of them is essential. A group decision should
be made for case disposition.

REPORTING

Reporting procedures will vary from place to place.
Both law enforcement bodies and social agencies may receive
child abuse reports. There should be clear understanding
by all what the requirements are in individual cases. Strict
legal interpretation may not always provide answers to specific questions. A good relationship is essential if coopera-
tive efforts are to succeed and jurisdictional disputes are
to be held to a minimum. The arrangement suggested by Kempe
and Helfer[12] (The Consortium) is the most detailed and comprehensive in the literature and is highly recommended. In
addition to organization in the hospital and the community,
their suggested development of parent groups for mutual aid
is superbly treated.

SUPPORT

Child abuse, although an ugly reminder of poorly controlled impulses of human behavior, needs to be brought out
of the closet. Failure to recognize trauma of this sort for
what it is, may be the result of parochial interest in medical technology, an aversion to admission of acting-out behavior present below the surface in all of us, or just too
little understanding of the implications of abuse. Whatever
the cause, we have an obligation to children as doctors to

produce the best possible environment for their growth and
development. We have many facts. We have many suggestions
about how to arrange for prevention of the fusion of forces
known to produce the explosion of violence. Our charge now
is to broaden, through education and community organization,
our capacity to act rationally and reduce the incidence of
the battered child syndrome.

REFERENCES

1. Caffey J: Multiple fractures in the long bones of in-
    fants suffering from chronic subdural hematoma. Amer
    J Roentgen 56:163, 1946

2. Cameron JM: The battered baby syndrome. The Practi-
    tioner 209:302, 1972

3. Dine MS: Tranquilizer poisoning: An example of child
    abuse. Pediatrics 36:782, 1965

4. Galdston R: Unpublished manuscript.

5. Gil D: Violence Against Children. Cambridge, Harvard
    University Press, 1970

6. Gregg GS, Elmer E: Infants injuries: Accident or
    abuse? Pediatrics 44:434, 1969

7. Harcourt B, Hopkins D: Opthalmic manifestations of the
    battered baby syndrome. BMJ 3:398, 1971

8. Helfer RE, Kempe CH: The Battered Child. Chicago,
    University of Chicago Press, 1968

9. Jackson G: Child abuse syndrome: The cases we miss.
    BMJ 2:756, 1972

10. Kempe CH, et al: The battered child syndrome. JAMA
    181:17, 1962

11. Kempe CH, Helfer RE: Helping the Battered Child and
    His Family. Philadelphia, Lippincott, 1972

12. Klein M, Stern L: Low birth weight and the battered
    child. Amer J Dis Child 122:15, 1971

13. Mushin AS: Occular damage in the battered baby syn-
    drome. BMJ 3:402, 1971

14. Silverman FN: The roentgen manifestations of unrecog-
    nized skeletal trauma in infants. Amer J Roentgen 69:
    413, 1953

15. Simons B, Downs EF, Hurster MM: Child abuse: Epide-
    miologic study of medically reported cases. New York
    J Med 66:2783, 1966

16. Toffler A: Future Shock. New York, Random House, 1970

CHAPTER 6

Prescribing

NAOMI BAUMSLAG and
EDWARD B. SILBERSTEIN

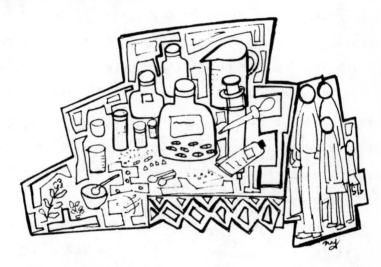

POINTS IN PRESCRIBING

THE PATIENT EXPECTS relief from the complaint and the doctor may be rated according to the effectiveness of the therapeutic regime. On the other hand patients tend to equate "good medicine" with drugs, and a doctor who fails to prescribe medicine may be judged as a "bad" doctor. Where relevant, take time out to explain why medication is not required or may even be harmful. Patients who have frequented hospital clinics for years make a fetish of pill taking and it is sometimes difficult to deprive such a

patient of his therapy or to change the regime, but don't
feel that you must prescribe. If practical, substitute a
diet for a useless pill, but don't prescribe placebos.

Once the problem is ascertained some plan must be implemented and therapy instituted. If tablets are to be used
it is necessary to know the strength supplied by the manufacturers. The Physician Desk Reference (PDR) carries this
information.[9] Make sure that you give the patient enough
tablets to treat the disease or to last until he needs to
return to the clinic or your office. In the case of a hospital patient make sure that the dispensary will issue the
quantity prescribed. Habit forming drugs should be dispense
in small quantities, e.g. barbiturates. Warn the mother who
is on dangerous drugs to keep the bottle in a safe place.
Explain the consequences of failing to do so. Even "safe"
tablets are potentially lethal, e.g. aspirin. Fatal overdosage can occur if the drug is not kept out of reach, is
stored in the wrong bottle (e.g. Coca-Cola bottle), or if
the patient is kept ignorant of the consequences of overdosage or fails to comprehend the instructions.

When prescribing ointments and creams, write the formul
as a percentage and state how it is to be applied. Always
caution the patient, if the lotion stains, to take the neces
sary precautions to avoid permanent damage to clothing or
embarrassing stains, e.g. vaginal suppositories. Always

write the percentage of active ingredients used in <u>solutions</u>
as they too come in different strengths.

DOSAGE AND OTHER CONSIDERATIONS

The age and condition of the person may modify the prescription. Renal and hepatic disease may be an indication
for reduced dosage. Medications for children are prescribed
usually as milligrams per meter squared (M^2). With infants
and children it is better to prescribe liquid formulations.
Pills can be more difficult to swallow whereas a sweet
tasting syrup base can help achieve cooperation. Make sure
that the medication prescribed has not expired and that
other requirements are also fulfilled. Penicillin V mixture
when in solution should be refrigerated; Chlorpheniramine
Maleate (Chlor-Trimeton) syrup should be kept out of the
light. Parents should be warned about the danger of accidental poisoning from ingestion of substances such as aspirin,
ferrous sulfate, (ferrous sulfate tablets can be mistaken
for chocolate colored M & M's.) All medication should be
kept out of reach of children in "child-proof" bottles.

The elderly frequently need to be supervised. Forget-
fulness or poor vision may lead to under or overdosage, particularly for regularly used drugs such as insulin. Make
certain that the patient can read and understands numbers
before giving the therapy. Also check the patient's dietary
habits. Alcohol potentiates the effects of many drugs, e.g.

barbiturates, diphenylhydantoin, etc.

In some cases the whole family may be required to take the medication, e.g. malaria or treatment of pinworm. If pyrvinium (Povan) is used in the treatment of pinworms[7] (Enterobius vermicularis), give as a single dose to each member of the family. Caution the patient about the unusual symptoms or side effects of the drug. Pyrvinium colors the stool bright red and if vomiting occurs on this regime, the bright red vomitus can be frightening if the patient has not been forewarned. Similarly if patients on Methyldopa (Aldomet) allow urine to stand before the toilet is flushed, it may develop a golden brown to deep red color, a rare complication, which may be mistaken for hematuria. However with Pyridium the urine is always a deep orange and the person taking the medicine must always be warned.

COST

For the most part generic drugs are less expensive than brand name or proprietary drugs. Also the active principle may be available as a number of compounds. Ferrous sulfate tablets are very cheap. Ferrous gluconate is much more expensive. The quality of the preparation is important and sometimes brand name drugs are of a higher quality and price versus quality must then be considered.

Tell the patient what medicine you are prescribing. Have the pharmacist put the name of the drug on the label so

that during a long illness similar pill boxes or mixtures
aren't confused. If necessary, the patient can obtain a re-
fill from you by telephone. Remember when prescribing pills
or mixtures for patients with chronic disease that pill
taking may be a cause of anxiety. Anxious patients tend to
watch the clock, so where possible reassure them and allow
some flexibility on the time of administration. If an adequate blood level can be obtained by medication twice a day,
do not prescribe t.i.d. It may mean that a child is given
added anxiety or embarrassment at school. A nurse may not
be available and mother might have to go to school every
lunch time. It is essential that you ascertain when prescribing:

1.   Is it necessary?

2.   What added strain am I imposing
     that could be avoided?

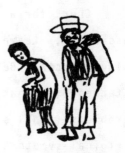

3.   Age (elderly and young often
     require special consideration
     when the dosage is calculated.

Try not to interrupt the daily schedule but let the medication be given so it coincides with important activities,
e.g. sleeping, eating, etc.

In prescribing one or many types of medications for
long term therapy make sure the family has some method of
cross checking to see that the required dose has been taken

or administered. A number of pills taken at a regular time
each day requires strong motivation and regulation. A crisis
could make it difficult to remember. When accidental omis-
sion of a single dose may result in a serious problem for
the patient, it is advisable to tell the family to make a
chart with times and dates and let the therapy be signed for
each time it is given.

Finally, when the patient's life depends on getting or
avoiding certain drugs, prescribe a bracelet. These are
easily obtainable. Epileptics, diabetics or patients with
drug allergy should wear such a bracelet or carry a card.
It can be life saving.

BEWARE OF THE THERAPEUTIC POISON

Check for a history of <u>allergy</u> or <u>sensitivity</u>. This is
essential. Learn to know the drugs you prescribe and their
side effects. Bear in mind that so called innocuous substances (such as antacids) are capable of producing other
problems (renal stones), sometimes more severe than the
original symptoms. Drugs should only be used continuously
under very well defined circumstances. In addition, certain
drugs that are administered to produce one effect, may produce another (anxiety states produced by some tranquilizers).
Alert patients of any untoward side effects (ataxia with
diphenylhydantoin) and warn them to call if worried or something unusual happens.

The use of drugs in pregnancy may pose special problems. Both the mother and fetus must be considered. The infant at the breast is also vulnerable if the mother is nursing. Lead poisoning has occurred in the newborn, where the mother was consuming large quantities of "moonshine" made in a lead lined battery.[8] The same effects can be produced by indiscriminate use of drugs in pregnancy. Thalidomide is one well-known teratogenic agent, but there may be more iatrogenic drug effects than are currently recognized.[2,10]

HOW TO WRITE A PRESCRIPTION[3]

Latin is no longer used in prescriptions. You will save the patient money if you get into the habit of prescribing generic names rather than trade names. Medications are generally prescribed in milligram or gram amounts per pill. Standard prescription pads are available. These have a space to fill in the date, name of clinic, patient's name, age, address and unit number.

(1) Under this information write the R_x symbol (recipe). The name of the drug should be written next to this and preferably should be printed. Indicate on the same line the concentration of the solution or the quantity of drugs.

(2) On the next line under R_x, you can write Disp., an abbreviation for "dispense" or simply state the amount of drug which you wish the patient to receive. This

will be recorded as the number of pills or the volume
of milliliters to be dispensed. For reference, one
teaspoon contains 5 ml., and one tablespoon contains
15 ml.

(3) On the third line of the prescription form, write the
abbreviation Sig. which is short for signa, the Latin
for "Label". This provides instructions for the patient
on how he is to take the medication. On the prescription abbreviations are generally used, e.g. 3 tabs.,
t.i.d., or 1 tsp. q. 4h. On the lower left of the
prescription indicate the frequency with which the
prescription may be refilled. If the drug is to be
used only externally, should be shaken well before
using, or is a poison when taken internally, such facts
must be stated. Avoid the phrase "Take as directed".

All prescriptions must be signed by a state licensed
physician. Narcotics cannot be dispensed without a narcotics
license number supplied by the Bureau of Narcotics and Dangerous Drugs.

The drugs given during pregnancy and lactation must be
carefully screened.[1] If in doubt, contact the Local Poison
Center to ascertain the potential hazards to the fetus. It
may be advisable to analyze the mother's milk if she is
nursing. If suppositories are used, the absorption factors
must be considered.

Sample Prescription

```
┌─────────────────────────────────────────────────────────┐
│                        Date                               │
│                        Patient's Name                     │
│                        Age                                │
│                        Patient's Address                  │
│                        Unit No.                           │
│ R_x:     Ferrous Sulfate o/300                            │
│ Disp:  100 tabs.                                          │
│ Sig:   1 tab. t.i.d. w/meals                              │
│ Label Refill X3                                           │
│                                                           │
│                        _____M.D.       │
│                        Narcotic No._____            │
└─────────────────────────────────────────────────────────┘
```

When using several drugs, make sure that they don't counteract or augment each other's effects (e.g. tetracyclines potentiate the effects of warfarin; phenobarbital decreases the effects of digitoxin).[12] If a conservative method such as diet will work, don't add a drug as the complications may be worse than the difficulty of dietary control. On the other hand be aware of the effect of certain foods (e.g. cheese may well precipitate a hypertensive crisis in a patient on a mono-amine oxidase inhibitor). Avoid appeasing the patient. To prescribe penicillin for influenze or any other viral infection is therapeutically unethical even if the patient demands a "shot". Find the most pleasant manner to administer the medicine, e.g. Vitamin C by injection is very painful, but oral Vitamin C is convenient,

effective and easier to administer. Save the patient unnecessary journeys by ensuring that he has sufficient medication for the prescribed period.

Drug Dosage

The individual variations to drug response of diphenylhydantoin, phenobarbitone, digoxin, quinidine, and salicy-
lates just to mention a few have been found to differ widely
in individual patients.[4] The "usual dose" of most potent
drugs "accomplishes little in some persons, and causes
serious toxicity in others and is fully satisfactory in few".
It is suggested that clinical impression and blood drug
levels should be viewed together in adjusting the dose. Considerable pressure is exerted on physicians to try out new
drugs and samples are constantly made available. It is
essential to critically but objectively weigh the value of
new drugs. Patients are individuals and the therapy should
fit the patient. Read the literature critically.[5,6] The resu
of a drug trial conducted on 100 men in a prison does not
necessarily reflect your patient's response to the same
drug. Learn to read graphs and interpret results scientifically. Do not hesitate to ask a competent physician or
colleague in the field for a second opinion.

Clearly instruct the patient as to how to take the medicine. Do not give written instructions to a person who cannot read, or to a foreigner not well versed in English.

Explain carefully and ask the patient to repeat your instructions if necessary.

Before you attribute side effects to a drug make sure the medication is being taken as prescribed. Bad taste or large pills may be reasons for patients discontinuing the medication. Long term usage of drugs should be prescribed with caution and the patient should be regularly evaluated to avoid other serious side effects of the drug. Stimulant drugs in hyperactive children have caused retardation of growth.[11]

Mistakes are more likely the longer the treatment, the more often the drug has to be taken and the greater the number of drugs to be taken. When medicines are prescribed you are giving instructions about a way of life and for compliance, maximum cooperation is needed on both sides.

REFERENCES

1. Arena JM: Contamination of the ideal food. Nutrition
    Today 5:2, 1970

2. D'Arcy DF, Griffin JP: Iatrogenic Diseases. London,
    Oxford University Press, 1972

3. Goodman LS, Gilman, AZ: Pharmacological Basis of Thera-
    peutics. Fourth edition. New York, MacMillan, 1970

4. Koch-Weser J: Serum drug concentrations as therapeutic
    guides. New Eng J of Med 287:227, 1972

5. Lionel NDW, Herxheimer A: Assessing reports of thera-
    peutic trials. Brit Med J 3:637, 1970

6. The Medical Letter. New Rochelle, The Medical Letter
    Inc.

7. Most H: Drug therapy: Common parasitic infections of
    man. New Eng J of Med 287:495, 1972

8. Palmisano PA, Sneed RC, Cassady G: Untaxed whisky and
    fetal lead exposure. J Ped 75:869, 1969

9. PDR. New Jersey, Medical Economics Inc., 1972

10. Rowe WS: Iatrogenic disease. Med J of Australia 2:
    560, 1969

11. Safer D, Allen R, Barr E: Depression of growth in
    hyperactive children on stimulant drugs. New Eng J
    Med 287:217, 1972

12. Solomon HM, Abrams WB: Interaction between digoxin and
    other drugs in man. Amer Ht J 83:277, 1972

Nutrition

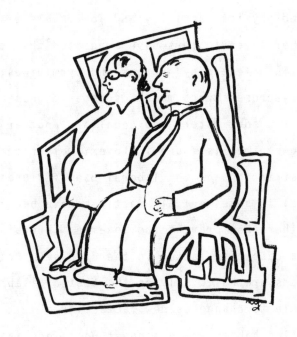

HUMAN NUTRITION SHOULD not be equated with calories,
weight and tables only. These are measures used
to modify specific diseases as scientifically as possible
and do not take into consideration the cultural factors
or geographic variations in food content. Although it is
essential that the physician be firm in prescribing a diet,
he must be aware that dietary regimes are constantly under
revision. Not only is the vitamin content of the diet

important, but the trace metal content must also be considere
Blood cholesterol and triglycerides may be used as markers in
the treatment of coronary artery disease. The factors that
protect farm laborers against heart disease may be strenuous
sustained physical activity and low levels of responsibility.
Many other investigators have suggested that coronary artery
disease is affected by purines and pyrmidines; carbohydrates
such as sucrose; trace metals such as magnesium, cadmium,
lithium (in soft water) and cobalt.[4] Another example of
changing regimes is found in toxemia of pregnancy. Stringent
salt restriction and the liberal use of diuretics (a vogue
or ritual in some medical practices have been shown to aggra-
vate rather than prevent the toxemia. Protein malnutrition
may be a causative factor in the disease. Prescribed special diets are based only on the best available information
and liable to change as new facts emerge.

Eating habits are dependent upon food availability,
individual economic resources, method of food preparation,
food storage and religious or tribal taboos and customs.
Most people eat at scheduled times rather than when they are
hungry. The food may be self-prepared, or it may come processed from a number of vending machines - hot dogs, hambur-
gers and pop. But the variation in feeding also takes other
forms. A vegetarian does not eat meat, meat products, fish
or fowl. Seventh day adventists and Hindus do not eat meat

or fish products either for religious reasons. A study of
Seventh Day Adventists has shown that the incidence of coronary artery disease and cancer is low among this group.[19]
Vegans eat no meat products at all excluding eggs, milk and
cheese from their diet. Vitamin B_{12} deficiency is more common in this group.

In America infants may be bottle fed and overdosed with
excessive calories, vitamins, and iron supplements. This
results in fat babies. Taitz et al[15] have shown that overfeeding the newborn produces obese adolescents and thus
introduces a high risk group for coronary artery disease and
hypertension. It is well documented that the highly refined
diets of the affluent western society are associated with
ulcerative colitis, celiac disease, diverticulitis and
cholelithiasis (gall stones).[12] On the other hand, protein -
calorie deficient diets give rise to kwashiorkor and marasmus - common in the underdeveloped countries but certainly
not unheard of in our affluent society.

An dietary habit practiced for years without thought,
may prove difficult to break and its background requires
sympathy and understanding on the part of the physician.

Eating is a way of life adapted to a particular geogra-
phy and culture and changing that way to a "better nutrition"
may bring many problems, e.g. in Malaya despite nutritionists'
urgings young children are not given fish (a good source of

protein) because Malayan mothers believe it produces worms.[6]
Africans newly subjected to "urbanization" which includes
new dietary habits, are becoming increasingly prone to coronary artery disease in areas where the disease was relatively
unknown.[13] In the Western Arctic, Eskimos relatively free
of diabetes in previous years are now showing a marked increase in the prevalence of the disease. Eskimos also show
an increase in atherosclerosis and dental caries attributed
to their new food habits.[12] Their consumption of sugar and
flour have increased markedly while their meat intake and
activity have been reduced. Campbell's rule[2] is that a
marked increase of diabetes morbidity in various population
groups follows after about 20 years of westernized diets
(where the annual sugar consumption exceeds 70 lbs.). The
"sugar climate" can be measured by DMFT rate (incidence of
total decayed, missing or filled teeth). The increasing
consumption of sugar in the affluent nations has been related
to increased secular growth acceleration. Sugar (sucrose)
uniquely supplies calories but no nutrients. Yudkin[20] has
advanced epidemiological evidence to show a correlation between sugar consumption and coronary artery disease. Diverticulitis coli is a disease of economically developed nations
who eat a diet in which the carbohydrate is refined. The
disease and its complications are an increasing problem in
Western countries and could be prevented if high residue
diets were consumed.

SPECIAL POINTS

IRON DEFICIENCY

Iron deficiency anemia is widespread in the USA and the iron needs of low income families and women of child-bearing age are not being met by the usual diet or by current iron fortification of bread and flour. The recommended daily allowance of the Food and Nutrition Board of the National Research Council for men is 10 mgs. and for women is 18 mgs. of iron. However, Crosby fears iron overload.[3] In South Africa 80% of autopsied Bantu cases have stainable iron in their livers due to their excessive intake of iron in Bantu beer made of degermed maize. In these cases the iron intake may be as high as 100-200 mgs. iron per day - quite in excess of the daily minimum requirements.[1] Furthermore, iron loss during pregnancy is about 680 mg. or close to 2.5 mg. per day. In iron deficiency anemia more than 2-20% iron is absorbed. The truth is we don't really know all the factors which influence iron absorption. It has been shown that calcium and phytates interfere with iron absorption. The balance between iron and other metals, e.g. lead, is not completely understood. Since the lead load of urban dwellers is higher than that of rural Americans, it is interesting to speculate that lead may interfere with iron absorption.

NUTRITION DURING PREGNANCY

Poor nutrition during pregnancy can affect mother and

infant. Severe maternal dietary deficiency could induce
malformations in the offspring.[16] Woodhill et al have shown
a relationship between the incidence of prematurity and
maternal dietary deficiency.[18]

The National Research Council states that there is no
justification for routine limitation of weight gain in pregnancy to less than 24 lbs. total.[8] Severe calorie restrictions are potentially harmful to both mother and fetus and
weight reduction of obese women should be undertaken inter-
partum and not during pregnancy. The report also cautions
restriction of salt and prescriptions of diuretics during
pregnancy. Furthermore, iodized salt is recommended for
areas where the soil is low in iodine in order to avoid cre-
tinism in the offspring.

PROTEIN CALORIE MALNUTRITION

When only the protein is deficient or absent but the
caloric intake is adequate, kwashiorkor occurs; this is common in malnourished children who develop edema, hair depig-
mentation, skin changes, failure of growth and are generally
apathetic and miserable. Marasmus is a consequence of almost
total starvation.

OBESITY

Obesity is a condition of excessive fat and it is perhaps the commonest dietary problem in this country. A person
is overweight if he is heavier than a given standard

(insurance company standards are often used) regardless of whether the distribution of weight is due to increased fat, muscle tissue or fluid. One method of measuring fat is called the "scientific pinch" using standardized calipers to measure subcutaneous fat-pads at specified places on the body.[14] There are two types of obesity.(1) Metabolic obesity - which is basically due to an endocrine abnormality. This is not common. (2) Regulatory obesity - which is due to a derangement of mechanism for food intake and/or energy expenditure. This by far constitutes the largest group. Talking to the patient and looking at him or her may be more informative than height and weight tables, especially in the case of children.[7]

CONSIDERATIONS WHEN PRESCRIBING A DIETARY REGIME

1.   Is it culturally acceptable?

      What is culturally acceptable often becomes palatable.
      Tacos, rice, pasta, mealie meal (pap), cassava bread,
      beans - are staple foods of different peoples prepared
      in specific ways and often difficult to eliminate from
      the diet. Folate deficiency in the African may be due
      to the fact that the only greens eaten are cooked for
      prolonged periods thus destroying folic acid content.
      In such instances it is easier to provide folic acid
      orally as tablets than to ask the people to buy and
      eat greens.

(2) Is it palatable?

The appearance of the food and its taste also affect
digestion and absorption. As one patient aptly put it
"The dietician asked me to eat cauliflower and liver.
How can I? - I am not a rabbit! And as for liver I
don't like it!" During World War II Western prisoners
in Japanese camps had to eat rice as the main, and often
only, meal. At first they all lost weight, developed
diarrhea and edema; but after a few months they started
gaining weight on the diet. When bread became available
after the war, they found that they could only eat a
little even though relished, without developing indigestion.[17]

3. Is anything interfering with absorption or utilization?

Rule out parasitic infestations or malabsorption syn-
dromes (as in pernicious anemia). Vegetables such as
cabbage and turnips, in large amounts, may be goitro-
genic.

4. How difficult is it to implement the changes?

Even if the patient is willing, if the diet imposes
hardship on the family and marked restrictions on a
way of life, the patient won't be able to follow it.
Persons living in hotels or travelling a lot may have
added problems.

5.   Is it economically feasible?

6.   Activity and exercise?

Assess the needs in terms of occupation and activity.

7.   Are there any added needs?

During pregnancy a woman needs an additional 300 calories per day and during lactation it has been estimated that 1000 calories per day are required in addition to those normally ingested.   Children need more calories than the elderly.[9]

8.   Age, weight, fat, height have all been used as parameters for controlling dietary intake.   However, it is most important to remember that you are prescribing a change in life style and it has to have the patient's acceptance.   Take care to have the dietician explain carefully what the regime involves and if the diet doesn't achieve its objectives try to find out why. There is no point in shouting at the patient or refusing to see him until he loses weight.   Punitive action of this sort adds further to the plight of the patient.

REFERENCES

1. Bothwell TH, Seftel HC, Jacobs P, Baumslag N: Iron
    overload in Bantu subjects: Studies on the availability
    of iron in Bantu beers. Jour Clin Nutrition 14:47, 1964

2. Cleave TL, Campbell GD, Painter NS: Diabetes Coronary
    Thrombosis and the Saccharine Disease. Bristol, John
    Wright and Sons Ltd, 1969

3. Crosby WH: Iron enrichment: One's food, another's
    poison. Arch Intern Med 126:911, 1970

4. Diet and coronary artery disease. BMJ 3:539, 1972
    (Editorial)

5. The Dietary Management of Hyperlipoproteinemia - A
    Handbook for Physicians. Washington, U.S. Public Health
    Service, 1969

6. Gifft HH, Washborn MB, Harrison GG: Nutrition, Behavior
    and Change. Englewood Cliffs, Prentice-Hall, Inc., 1972

7. Mayer J: Overweight: Causes, Costs and Control.
    Englewood Cliffs, Prentice-Hall, 1968

8. National Research Council: Maternal Nutrition and the
    Course of Human Pregnancy. Washington, National Academy
    of Sciences, 1968

9. National Research Council: Recommended Dietary Allow-
    ances. Seventh edition. Washington, National Academy
    of Sciences, 1968

10. Obesity and Health. Washington, U.S. Public Health
    Service Publication, No. 1485, 1967

11. Painter NS, Burkitt DP: Diverticular disease of the
    colon: A deficiency disease of western civilization.
    BMJ 2:450, 1971

12. Schaefer O: When the Eskimo comes to town. Nutrition
    Today 6:8, 1971

13. Seftel HC, Kew MC: Myocardial infarction in Johannes-
    burg Bantu. S. Afr Med J 44:8, 1970

14. Seltzer CC, Mayer J: A simple criterion of obesity.
    Postgraduate Medicine 38:A101, 1965

15. Taitz LS: Infantile overnutrition among artificially
    fed infants in the Sheffield region. BMJ 1:315, 1971

16. Warkany J: Congenital malformations induced by maternal
    nutritional deficiency. J Pediatrics 25:476, 1944

17. Williams C: Social aspects of nutrition. Matrix of
    Medicine. Edited by Mellison. Pitman Medical Publi-
    cations, 1958

18. Woodhill IM, Van der Berg AS, Burke BS, Stare FJ:
    Nutrition studies of pregnant Australian women: 1.
    Maternal nutrition in relation to toxemia of pregnancy
    and physical condition of the infant at birth. Am J
    Obstet Gynec 70:987, 1955

19. Wynder EL, Lemon FR, Bross IJ: Cancer and coronary
    artery disease among Seventh Day Adventists. Cancer
    12:1016, 1959

20. Yudkin J, Edelman J, Hough L: Sugar. London, Butter-
    worths, 1971

RECOMMENDED SOURCE BOOKS

1. Food: Yearbook of Agriculture 1959. Washington, U.S.
   Department of Agriculture, 1959

2. Underwood EG: Trace Elements in Human and Animal Nutrition. Third edition. New York, Academic Press, 1972

3. Williams SR: Nutrition and Diet Therapy. Saint Louis,
   Mosby, 1969

CHAPTER 7

Diet and the Diabetic

JOHN K. DAVIDSON

THE UNIVERSITY GROUP Diabetes Program study[1,2] has forced a re-examination of the philosophy of the treatment of maturity-onset diabetes mellitus. For approximately fifteen years, there has been almost unbridled enthusiasm among physicians and patients for the use of sulfonylureas and phenformin as treatments of choice, so that approximately one and one-half million Americans are now being treated with oral hypoglycemic agents. It is now obvious that these drugs are not satisfactory substitutes for proper diet therapy and weight reduction. It is also clear that insulin therapy is not a satisfactory substitute for diet therapy and weight reduction in this group of patients, although insulin therapy was not associated with an increased risk of cardiovascular death as was tolbutamide and phenformin therapy.

EDUCATION OF THE PATIENT

It is the responsibility of the physician and the allie
health personnel (nurse, dietitian, podiatrist, pharmacist,
social worker and laboratory technicians) who work with him
to teach the patient and his family everything that he needs
to know to optimally control diabetes. This includes the
objectives of treatment, diet, insulin therapy and side
effects of such therapy and how to treat them (especially
hypoglycemia), how to recognize and manage ketoacidosis,
how to test urine for glucose and acetone, the importance
of foot care and general hygienic measures, and the importance of regular follow-up by the physician, nurse and dieti
tian. (Diet manuals that may be useful in teaching the
patient are listed at the end of this chapter).

PRESCRIBING THE DIET

The diabetic diet may differ from the family's general
diet in four ways: (1) foods containing concentrated carbohydrates are restricted and sweetened foods are omitted;
(2) the amount of food eaten is measured or accurately esti
mated; (3) food is prepared in such ways that the content
of a serving in food exchanges is known; and (4) meals, and
between-meal snacks, if prescribed, are eaten at the same
times each day. Special or dietetic foods are not required
and should be carefully avoided because they contain a large
number of calories and/or sugar alcohols that are converted

to glucose in the body.

A prescription for a diabetic diet contains: (1) the number of calories; (2) the content in grams of protein, carbohydrate and fat; and (3) the fractional caloric and carbohydrate distribution into meals (and snacks if needed) each day.

First, estimate the patient's ideal body weight, and then calculate the number of calories the patient should eat each day to attain (or maintain) this weight. Then weigh the patient at regular intervals to determine whether or not he is eating the correct number of calories. If the weight pattern indicates that the patient is eating too much food, decrease the number of calories in the prescription. If the weight pattern indicates that the patient is eating too little food, increase the number of calories in the prescription.

ESTIMATION OF OPTIMAL CALORIC INTAKE

Basal Calories: The average adult uses about 10 calories per pound of ideal body weight at complete bed rest.

Activity Calories: These are estimated by adding calculated percentages to basal calories. For mild (sedentary) activity add 30%; for moderate activity add 50%; and for strenuous activity add 100%.

Growth Calories: Pregnant women require additional calories to assure a normal rate of growth. They are classified by their body weight at the beginning of pregnancy, and the caloric prescription written accordingly: (1) if of ideal body weight, about 2000 calories per day are prescribed; (2) if 15% above ideal body weight, about 1800 calories per day are prescribed; (3) if underweight, about 2200 calorie per day are prescribed.

Patients who are overweight have an excess number of calories stored in their adipose tissue. These calories may be depleted and the excess weight lost by having the patient eat fewer calories than his estimated basal and activity caloric need. Thus a caloric deficit of 500 calori per day will result in a weight loss of about one pound per week, while a caloric deficit of 1000 calories per day will result in a weight loss of about two pounds per week. Similar daily caloric excesses will result in a weight gain of one or two pounds per week, respectively.

CALORIE CONTENT: PROTEIN, CARBOHYDRATE AND FAT

One gram of protein provides 4 calories. One gram of fat provides 9 calories. One gram of carbohydrate equals 4 calories. For adults the calories are divided as follows: one-half gram (or more if the patient desires) of protein per pound of ideal body weight (with a minimum of 60 grams); the remaining calories are about equally divided between carbohydrate and fat, although in reduction diets and hyperliproteinemia diets, fats (especially saturated fats and

cholesterol) are disproportionally restricted. For pregnant
women, the calories are divided into about 20% protein, 40%
carbohydrate and 40% fat.

FRACTIONAL DISTRIBUTION INTO MEALS

It is convenient to divide the daily caloric prescription into tenths. Thus, each meal usually contains about
2/10, 3/10 or 4/10 of the day's food allowance, and each
snack usually contains about 1/10 fractional distribution.
Since the fractional distribution into calories and carbohydrate may not always accurately translate into a specified
number of food exchanges, a deviation of up to 10% from the
prescribed fractional distribution is considered satisfactory. The fractional distribution should be adjusted to
minimize the possibilities of hypoglycemia or hyperglycemia.
Thus, if post-breakfast hyperglycemia occurs when 3/10 of
the calories are eaten at breakfast, breakfast calories
should be reduced to 2/10. When hypoglycemia occurs before
the next meal, an additional 1/10 should be added to the
preceding meal, or a snack of 1/10 should be added prior to
the time hypoglycemia is prone to occur. All patients on
insulin therapy should have a bedtime snack.

OTHER ADJUSTMENTS IN DIET

Since the diabetic diet is nutritionally adequate, no
supplementary vitamins or minerals are needed unless the
physician prescribes them. During pregnancy, supplementary

vitamins are usually prescribed, and the calcium intake
should be 1.5 grams per day. After the 20th week of pregnancy, sodium chloride intake may be limited to 5 grams (2
grams sodium) per day. In the presence of congestive heart
failure or hypertension, the sodium intake may be restricted
to 2 grams per day (see Table 7.2). In the presence of
hyperlipoproteinemia, saturated fats and cholesterol may be
limited (see Table 7.3).

FOOD EXCHANGES

Different types of food that are allowed on diabetic
diets have been divided into six groups, or exchange lists:

Milk	Bread
Vegetable	Meat
Fruit	Fat

The number of calories, and the amount of protein, carbohydrate and fat in each food exchange within a group (but not
between groups) are approximately equal. Thus, within any
food group a specified amount of one food may be exchanged
for a specified amount of another food (1/2 banana may be
exchanged for 1 orange, 1/2 cup of grits may be exchanged
for 1 slice of bread, etc). However, 1/2 cup of grits cannot be exchanged for 1 orange.

Either the physician or dietitian (or her surrogate)
must translate the dietary prescription into servings of
various foods that are allowed. The diet should be adapted
to the patient's food preferences to the greatest possible

extent. However, it must be clearly recognized, and repeatedly emphasized, that for the majority of patients, the diabetic diet necessitates a departure from long-established
and deeply ingrained eating habits. This is of critical
importance in the obese. It is easy to blame failure of
diet therapy on lack of patient motivation or cooperation;
the sad fact is that in the majority of cases, it is due to
failure of the physician to prescribe a proper diet and to
persist in his educational efforts until the patient's lifelong eating habits have been altered. Of course, the patient
must be repeatedly reminded that it is he and the one who
prepares his food who must implement the dietary prescription and assure its success. If the patient is a neurotic
or psychotic compulsive eater, group or individual psychotherapy should be undertaken.

Five examples of dietary prescriptions and their translation into food exchanges are given in Tables 7.4, 7.5,
7.6, 7.7 and 7.8. The six exchange lists are given in
Tables 7.9, 7.10, 7.11, 7.12, 7.13 and 7.14. Foods that
are allowed in reasonable amounts and foods that should be
avoided are listed in Table 7.15. Frequently used dietary
prescriptions are listed in Table 7.16.

Table 7.1
IDEAL WEIGHTS FOR MEN AND WOMEN
According to Height and Frame. Ages 25 and over.

Height (in shoes)	Weight in Pounds (in Indoor Clothing)		
	Small Frame	Medium Frame	Large Frame
Men			
5' 2"	112-120	118-129	126-141
3"	115-123	121-133	129-144
4"	118-126	124-136	132-148
5"	121-129	127-139	135-152
6"	124-133	130-143	138-156
7"	128-137	134-147	142-161
8"	132-141	138-152	147-166
9"	136-145	142-156	151-170
10"	140-150	146-160	155-174
11"	144-154	150-165	159-179
6' 0"	148-158	154-170	164-184
1"	152-162	158-175	168-189
2"	156-167	162-180	173-194
3"	160-171	167-185	178-199
4"	164-175	172-190	182-204
Women			
4'10"	92-98	96-107	104-119
11"	94-101	98-110	106-122
5' 0"	96-104	101-113	109-125
1"	99-107	104-116	112-128
2"	102-110	107-119	115-131
3"	105-113	110-122	118-134
4"	108-116	113-126	121-138
5"	111-119	116-130	125-142
6"	114-123	120-135	129-146
7"	118-127	124-139	133-150
8"	122-131	128-143	137-154
9"	126-135	132-147	141-158
10"	130-140	136-151	145-163
11"	134-144	140-155	149-168
6' 0"	138-148	144-159	153-173

Note: Prepared by the Metropolitan Life Insurance Company. Derived
primarily from data of the Build and Blood Pressure Study, 1959,
Society of Actuaries.

Table 7.2

SUGGESTIONS FOR SODIUM RESTRICTED DIETS

Avoid salt, soda, and baking powder. Salt should not be used in the preparation of food or added at the table.

Avoid other foods in exchanges as listed below:

Milk	Commercial buttermilk. Limit other milk to 1 quart per day.
Vegetable	Sauerkraut
Fruit	No restrictions
Bread	Cornbread, salted crackers, pork and beans, quick-cooking or instant cereals, self-rising flour, meal, biscuits
Meat	Ham, wieners, bologna, luncheon meats, cured meats, creamed cottage cheese, cheese, all meats canned with salt, peanut butter
Fat	Bacon, fat back, sausage, olives, commercial salad dressings, salted nuts
Foods Allowed in Reasonable Amount (page 20)	Bouillon, celery salt, onion salt, garlic salt, monosodium glutamate, catsup, mustard, soy sauce, Worcestershire sauce, Shasta, Fresca.
Combination Foods	Most foods on the Combined Foods List (pages 25–26) contain salt. Check package labels carefully for salt content before using any of them.

Tables on this and following pages are reproduced with permission from John K. Davidson and Mary R. Goldsmith: _Diabetes Guidebook, Diet Section._ 1972.

Table 7.3

Dietary prescription for a 40-year old diabetic adult male office worker, 69 inches tall, medium frame, weight 160 pounds, who takes 38 units NPH insulin each morning before breakfast. He is moderately active physically.

(a) Ideal Body Weight = $106 + 9(6) = 160$ pounds
(b) Estimated caloric need
    (1) Basal calories = 160 pounds x 10 calories per pound =   1600 Calories
    (2) Activity calories = + 50% =   + 800 Calories

                                                            2400 Calories

(c) Division into grams of   Protein   Carbohydrate   Fat
                             80 gm.   260 gm.   116 gm.

(d) Division into meals and a snack
     3/10 breakfast   3/10 lunch   3/10 supper   1/10 bedtime snack

TRANSLATION INTO FOOD EXCHANGES

FOOD	Total For Day	Grams Pro	Grams Cho	Grams Fat	Total Calories	Distribution B	L	AS	S	HS
Milk	2	16	24	16	304	1				1
Vegetables	3	3	15	–	72		1		2	
Fruit	4	–	40	–	160	2	1		1	
Bread	12	24	180	–	816	3	4		4	1
Meat	5	35	–	25	365	1	2		2	
Fat	15	–	–	75	675	5	4		6	
Total		78	259	116	2392					
Fractional Distribution						3/10	3/10		3/10	1/10

Table 7.4

Dietary prescription for a 25-year old diabetic male bricklayer whose physical activity is strenuous. He is 71 inches tall, of small frame, and weighs 140 pounds. He takes 45 units NPH insulin each morning before breakfast. He likes meat and can afford to buy it.

(a) Ideal Body Weight = 106 + 11(6) − 10% = 172 - 17 pounds = 155 pounds

(b) Estimated caloric need

    (1) Basal Calories = 155 pounds x 10 calories per pound =   1550 Calories

    (2) Activity Calories = +100% =   +1550 Calories

    (3) Growth Calories to gain about 1 pound each week =   + 500 Calories

    3600 Calories

(c) Division into grams of Protein   Carbohydrate   Fat
                         160 gm   370 gm.   165 gm.

    (only 78 gm protein required to provide 1/2 gm/lb I.B.W., but he likes meat so

    1 gm+/lb. I.B.W. was prescribed)

(d) Division into meals and a snack

    3/10 breakfast   3/10 lunch   3/10 supper   1/10 bedtime snack

This dietary prescription will be revised when he reaches his I.B.W. of 155 pounds to contain 3100 calories/day.

TRANSLATION INTO FOOD EXCHANGES

FOOD	Total For Day	Grams Pro	Grams Cho	Grams Fat	Total Calories	B	L	AS	S	HS
Milk	3	24	36	24	456	1	1			1
Vegetables	5	5	25	–	120		2		3	
Fruit	5	–	50	–	200	2			2	1
Bread	17	34	255	–	1156	5	6		5	1
Meat	14	98	–	70	1022	3	5		6	
Fat	14	–	–	70	630	4	4		4	2
Total		161	366	164	3584					
Fractional Distribution						3/10	3/10		3/10	1/10

Table 7.5

Dietary prescription for a 65-year old mildly diabetic female who is 61 inches tall, medium frame, and weighs 198 pounds. She is sedentary in her physical activity.

(a) Ideal Body Weight = 100 + 1(5) = 105 pounds

(b) Estimated caloric need

  (1) Basal calories = 105 pounds x 10 calories per pound =   1050 Calories

  (2) Activity calories = +30% =   + 315 Calories

                                                                  1365 Calories

  (3) Decrease caloric intake by 35% to lose about 1 pound each week

                                                                 — 477 Calories

                                                                  888 Calories

(c) Division into grams of   Protein   Carbohydrate   Fat
                              60 gm.   100 gm.   28 gm.

(d) Division into meals
     2/10 breakfast   4/10 lunch   4/10 supper

TRANSLATION INTO FOOD EXCHANGES

FOOD	Total For Day	Grams Pro	Grams Cho	Grams Fat	Total Calories	B	L	AS	S	HS
Milk, Skim	2 1/2	20	30	—	200	1	1/2		1	
Vegetables	2	2	10	—	48		1		1	
Fruit	3	—	30	—	120	1	1		1	
Bread	2	4	30	—	136		1		1	
Meat	5	35	—	25	365	1	2		2	
Fat	0	—	—	—						
Total		61	100	25	869					
Fractional Distribution						2/10	4/10		4/10	

Table 7.6

Dietary prescription for a 34-year old mildly diabetic female housewife who is 66 inches tall, weighs 173 pounds, is moderately active, and has a large frame.

(a) Ideal Body Weight = 100 +6(5) +10% for large frame = 143 pounds

(b) Estimated caloric need

    (1) Basal Calories = 143 pounds x 10 calories per pound =   1430 Calories

    (2) Activity calories = +50% =   + 715 Calories

                                                            2145 Calories

    (3) Decrease caloric intake by 30% to lose about 1.5 pounds each week

                                                          – 645 Calories

                                                          1500 Calories

(c) Division into grams of   Protein   Carbohydrate Fat

                              75 gm.   150 gm.   66gm.

(d) Division into meals

    3/10 breakfast   3/10 lunch 4/10 supper

TRANSLATION INTO FOOD EXCHANGES

FOOD	Total For Day	Grams Pro	Grams Cho	Grams Fat	Total Calories	B	L	AS	S	HS
Milk	2	16	24	16	304	1/2	1		1/2	
Vegetables	3	3	15	–	72		1		2	
Fruit	2	–	20	–	80	1			1	
Bread	6	12	90	–	408	2	2		2	
Meat	6	42	–	30	438	1	2		3	
Fat	4	–	–	20	180	2	1		1	
Total		73	149	66	1482					
Fractional Distribution						3/10	3/10		4/10	

Table 7.7

Dietary prescription for a 28-year old mildly diabetic female housewife (moderate activity) of medium frame who is 63 inches tall, weighs 118 pounds, and is 5 months pregnant. She has mild pedal edema and mild hypertension.

(a) Ideal Body Weight (non-pregnant) = $100 + 3(5) = 115$ pounds.

(b) Estimated caloric need (to gain 23 pounds during pregnancy) = 2000 calories

(c) Division into grams of protein (20%), carbohydrate (40%), and fat (40%)

      Protein   Carbohydrate   Fat

      100 gm.   200 gm.   89 gm.

(d) Division into meals and a snack

      3/10 breakfast   3/10 lunch   3/10 supper   1/10 bedtime snack

(e) The diet should contain 1.5 gm. calcium per day, sodium chloride intake should be limited to 5 gm. per day, and a multivitamin capsule should be prescribed each day.

TRANSLATION INTO FOOD EXCHANGES

FOOD	Total For Day	Grams Pro	Grams Cho	Grams Fat	Total Calories	Distribution B	L	AS	S	HS
Milk	4	32	48	32	608	1	1		1	1
Vegetables	3	3	15	–	72		1		2	
Fruit	5	–	50	–	200	2	1		1	1
Bread	6	12	90	–	408	2	2		2	
Meat	8	56	–	40	584	2	3		3	
Fat	3	–	–	15	135	1	1		1	
Total		103	203	87	2007					
Fractional Distribution						3/10	3/10		3/10	1/10

Table 7.8

MILK EXCHANGES – One exchange of milk contains 12 grams Carbohydrate, 8 grams Protein, 8 grams Fat, and 152 Calories.

Whole milk (Plain or homogenized)	1 cup
*Skim milk	1 cup
Evaporated milk (undiluted)	1/2 cup
Powdered whole milk	1/4 cup
*Powdered skim milk (non-fat dried milk)	1/4 cup
*Instant powdered skim milk (non-fat dried milk)	1/3 cup
*Buttermilk (made from skim milk)	1 cup
+Light'n Lively or One-Ten milk (1% fat)	1 cup
++2% Fortified milk (2% fat)	1 cup
Yogurt, plain (made with whole milk)	1 cup
+Yogurt, plain (made with skim milk)	1 cup

* If your diet calls for whole milk, you may substitute skim milk or buttermilk provided you add 1 1/2 fat exchanges for each cup of skim milk or buttermilk you use. Skim milk and buttermilk have the same food value as whole milk except they are lower in fat.

\+ If your diet calls for whole milk, you may use Light'n Lively, One-Ten milk, or yogurt made with skim milk in place of the whole milk. You will need to add 1 fat exchange to your meal for each cup substituted.

++ If your diet calls for whole milk, you may use 2% fat milk in place of the whole milk. You will need to add 1/2 fat exchange to your meal for each cup substituted.

   All milks cannot be listed, so check with your physician or dietitian about substituting any unlisted milk product that you wish to use.

One quart of milk contains approximately one gram of calcium.

Table 7.9

VEGETABLE EXCHANGES — Although some vegetables have been listed in the past as free foods, they do contain calories. In this manual, they have been divided into servings that average 5 grams carbohydrate, 1 gram protein, and 24 calories. Accordingly, the size serving is listed in 1 cup, 1/2 cup, or 1/4 cup amounts.

1 cup equals one serving	1/2 cup equals one serving	1/4 cup equals one serving
Asparagus	Artichoke	Green peas
Beans, string	Bamboo shoots	*Winter squash
Beans, wax	Beets	Mixed vegetables
Bean sprouts	*Beet greens	
Cabbage	*Broccoli	
Cauliflower	Brussels sprouts	
Celery	*Carrots	
*Chard	*Collards	
Chicory	*Dandelion greens	
Cucumbers	Eggplant	
Endive	*Kale	
Escarole	Mushrooms	
Lettuce	*Mustard greens	
Okra	Onions	
Pepper	*Poke salad	
Radishes	*Pumpkin	
Rhubarb	Rutabagas	
Sauerkraut	*Spinach	
Squash, summer	Tomatoes	
*Turnip greens	Tomato juice	
*Watercress	Turnips	
	Vegetable juice (V-8)	

* These vegetables contain a lot of vitamin A. Try to eat one of them every day.

Vegetables should be measured the way they are eaten—cooked or raw. Fat allowed on the diet may be used to season the vegetables. Vinegar and lemon juice may also be used for seasoning.

Vegetables may be cooked in bouillon or fat-free meat broth, if desired.

If you eat vegetables that have been cooked with fat meat, ham hock, oil, margarine, or butter, allow 1 fat exchange for each serving of vegetable eaten. This must be counted as part of your fat allowance.

Table 7.10

FRUIT EXCHANGES — One exchange of fruit contains 10 grams Carbohydrate and 40 Calories.

Fruit	Amount	Fruit	Amount
Apple (2" diameter)	1 small	Grapes	12
Apple juice	1/3 cup	Grape Juice	1/4 cup
Applesauce	1/2 cup	Honeydew Melon (7" diameter)	1/8
Apricots, fresh	2 medium	Mango	1/2 small
Apricots, dried or canned	4 halves	Nectarine	1 small
Banana	1/2 small	*Orange (2½" diameter)	1 small
Berries-Blackberries	1 cup	*Orange Juice	1/2 cup
Boysenberries	1 cup	Peach (2" diameter)	1 medium
Raspberries	1 cup	Peaches, canned	2 halves
Strawberries	1 cup	Pear (2" diameter)	1 small
Blueberries	2/3 cup	Pears, canned	2 halves
*Cantaloupe (6" diameter)	1/4	Pineapple	1/2 cup
Cherries	10 large	Pineapple Juice	1/3 cup
Cranberries	1 cup	Plums	2 medium
Dates	2	Prunes, dried	2 medium
Figs, fresh	2 large	Prune Juice	1/4 cup
Figs, dried	1 small	Raisins	2 tablespoons
Fruit Cocktail	1/2 cup	*Tangerine	1 large
*Grapefruit	1/2 small	Watermelon	1 cup
*Grapefruit Juice	1/2 cup		

Fruits may be fresh, dried, cooked, canned, or frozen without sugar.

Artificially-sweetened fruit is more expensive than water-packed fruit. It is not necessary to buy "diet" fruit. Read the label on the fruit to be sure it says "unsweetened" or "no sugar added."

*   These fruits are good sources of Vitamin C. Try to use one of them each day.

Table 7.11

BREAD EXCHANGES — One bread exchange contains 15 grams Carbohydrate, 2 grams Protein, and 68 Calories.

Bread

White, whole wheat, or rye,	1 slice
Biscuit (2" diameter)	1
Bagel	1/2
Bun, Hamburger (medium)	1/2
Wiener, (medium)	1/2
Cornbread (1 1/2" cube)	1 piece
Corn Muffin (2 1/2" diameter)	1/2
English Muffin	1/2
Roll (2" diameter)	1
Breadcrumbs	3 tablespoons
Matzoth (6" diameter)	1 piece

Crackers

Saltines (2" square)	5
Waverly wafers	5
Graham (2 1/2" square)	2
Oyster	20 or 1/2 cup
Soda crackers (2 1/2" square)	3
Ry-Krisp	4 small
Triscuits	4 small
Holland Rusk	2
Zwieback	2 small
Round, thin (1 1/2", Ritz, Hi Ho)	6
Pretzels, 3-ring	6

Cornstarch	2 tablespoons
Flour	2 1/2 tablespoons
Cereal, cooked	1/2 cup
(oatmeal, Cream of Wheat, farina)	
Dry	3/4 cup
(cornflakes, puffed wheat, etc.)	
Grits, rice (cooked)	1/2 cup
Noodles, spaghetti, macaroni (cooked)	1/2 cup

Potatoes

White (2" diameter)	1 small
White, mashed	1/2 cup
Sweet or yams	1/4 cup

Vegetables

Beans, dried, cooked	1/2 cup
(Pinto, navy, great northern)	
Peas, dried or fresh, cooked	1/2 cup
(Black-eyed, field, crowder, Lady, or split peas)	
Lima beans or butterbeans	1/2 cup
Corn	1/3 cup or 1/2 small ear
Popcorn, unbuttered	1 1/2 cups
Parsnips	1/2 cup
Succotash	1/3 cup
Pork and beans	1/4 cup
Baked beans	1/4 cup

Measure all foods on this list after they have been cooked. These foods should be cooked in water (salted if salt is permitted) and seasoned with allowed fat after they have been measured.

Table 7.12

MEAT EXCHANGES – One Meat exchange contains 7 grams Protein, 5 grams Fat, and 73 Calories.

Meat and poultry	.1 slice (4" x 2" x 1/4")
(beef, lamb, pork, liver, chicken, turkey)	
Fish	.1 slice (4" x 2" x 1/4")
(croaker, mullet, perch, snapper, or catfish)	
Salmon, tuna, crab, or lobster	1/4 cup
Sardines	3 medium
Shrimp or oysters	.5 small
Brains	1/2 cup
Egg	.1
Cheese	1 ounce slice
Cottage cheese	1/4 cup
Cold cuts	.1 slice
(bologna, lunch meat, minced ham)	
Canadian bacon	1 slice (2 1/2" diameter x 1/4")
Sousemeat	.1 slice (4" x 3" x 1/8")
Wieners (8-9 per pound)	1
Vienna sausage	2 medium
Peanut butter (limit to 1 serving per day. Omit 2 fat exchanges)	.2 tablespoons

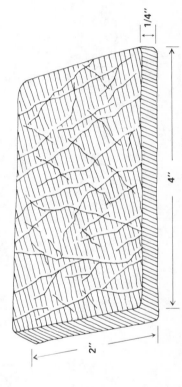

All excess fat should be cut from the meat before it is cooked. Meats may be baked in foil, broiled, boiled, roasted, or fried. Fat exchanges allowed on the diet must be used when the meat is fried. For example, if you eat a fried egg for breakfast, count it as 1 meat exchange and 1 fat exchange.

Table 7.13

FAT EXCHANGES — One fat exchange contains 5 grams Fat and 45 Calories.

Butter or oleomargarine	1 teaspoon
Breakfast bacon, crisp	1 slice
Bacon grease	1 teaspoon
Cracklins	1 heaping teaspoon
Cream, heavy	1 tablespoon
Cream, light	2 tablespoons
Half and Half	2 tablespoons
Cream, sour	2 tablespoons
Cream cheese	1 tablespoon
Fat back	See note below*
French dressing	1 tablespoon
Lard	1 teaspoon
Mayonnaise	1 teaspoon
Nuts	
Almonds	8 nuts
Brazil nuts	2 nuts
Cashews	5 nuts
Chestnuts	See note below**
Filberts	5 nuts
Hazelnuts	5 nuts
Hickory nuts	7 nuts
Macadamia	3 nuts
Pecans	6 halves
Peanuts	6 whole
Pistachio	20 nuts
Black walnuts	5 halves
English walnuts	6 halves
Oil, cooking	1 teaspoon
Olives	5 small
Shortening (Crisco, Snowdrift)	1 teaspoon
Avocado (4" diameter)	1/8

*All of the fat does not cook out of fatback when it is boiled or fried. For this reason, the amount to use when seasoning one serving of a vegetable depends on whether you eat the fatback or not. If you plan to eat the fatback, use a piece that is 1" x 1" x 1/4". If you eat only the vegetable, use a piece of fatback that is 2" x 1" x 1/2". Either will equal one fat exchange.

If you eat a slice of fried fatback, use a raw slice 6" x 2" x 1/4", fry very crisp, and drain on a paper towel. This equals 1 fat exchange.

**3 large chestnuts contain 9.3 grams carbohydrate and 0.3 grams fat and should be counted as 1 fruit exchange.

If you eat vegetables that have been cooked with fat meat, ham hock. oil, margarine, or butter, allow 1 fat exchange for each serving of vegetable eaten. This must be counted as part of your fat allowance.

If your diet does not allow fat exchanges, your vegetables must be cooked without fat. Bouillon or fat-free broth may be used.

The following foods are equal to 2 fat exchanges: 1/2 sausage patty (2 1/2" diameter). 1 link pork sausage (3" x 1/2" diameter), 1/4 cup boiled chitterlings ("chitlins").

Table 7.14

FOODS ALLOWED IN REASONABLE AMOUNTS

Black Coffee

Bouillon

Broth, fat-free

Condiments - salt, pepper, cinnamon, mustard, onion salt, garlic
  salt, celery salt, spices

Vinegar

Catsup - limit to 1 teaspoon per meal

Lemon juice

Gelatin, plain

D-Zerta gelatin

Pickles, sour and dill

Tea

Saccharin and other artificial sweeteners that do not contain
  sugar, lactose, or sorbitol

Vanilla and other flavoring extracts

Garlic

Mint leaf

Parsley

Diet drinks that do not contain sugar - Fresca, Diet Shasta, Tab

Postum - limit to 2 teaspoons

Cocoa - limit to 1 teaspoon

Soy sauce

Worcestershire sauce

FOODS THAT SHOULD BE AVOIDED

Sugar

Candy

Honey

Jam

Jelly

Jello

Pies

Cakes

Cookies

Dietetic foods that contain sugar, mannitol, sorbitol, or lactose-
  for example, dietetic ice cream, dietetic candy, or dietetic
  cookies

Ice cream, ice milk, sherbet

Sweets of any kind

Sweet rolls

Doughnuts

Chewing gum, regular and dietetic

Regular soft drinks

Diet soft drinks that contain sugar - for example, Diet Pepsi,
  Diet Rite, Diet Dr. Pepper

Alcoholic beverages - unless your physician specifically permits
  you to use them

Artificial sweeteners that contain lactose or sorbitol

Table 7.15

FREQUENTLY USED DIETARY PRESCRIPTIONS

DIET PRESCRIPTION					BREAKFAST					LUNCH						SUPPER						SNACK				
Calories	Pro. (gms)	CHO (gms)	Fat (gms)	Division	Milk	Fruit	Bread	Meat	Fat	Milk	Veg.	Fruit	Bread	Meat	Fat	Milk	Veg.	Fruit	Bread	Meat	Fat	Milk	Fruit	Bread	Meat	Fat
800	60	85	25	3/10, 3/10, 4/10	1 skim	–	1	1	–	1/2 skim	2	1	–	2	–	1 skim	1	–	1	2	–	–	–	–	–	–
1000	70	125	25	3/10, 3/10, 4/10	1 skim	1	1	1	–	1 skim	2	–	1	2	–	1 skim	1	2	1	2	–	–	–	–	–	–
1200	70	125	45	3/10, 3/10, 4/10	1 skim	1	1	1	2	1 skim	2	–	1	2	1	–	2	1	2	3	1	–	–	–	–	–
1500	70	150	70	3/10, 3/10, 3/10, 1/10	1/2	1	2	2	1	1	2	1	1	2	1	1/2	2	–	2	2	1	1	–	–	–	–
1800	80	180	85	3/10, 3/10, 3/10, 1/10	1	1	2	2	1	1/2	2	1	2	2	2	1/2	2	1	2	2	2	–	–	–	1	1
2000	90	200	95	3/10, 3/10, 3/10, 1/10	1	2	2	2	2	1/2	2	1	2	2	3	1/2	2	1	2	2	3	1/2	–	1	1	1
2200	90	220	105	3/10, 3/10, 3/10, 1/10	1	1	3	2	3	–	2	1	3	2	4	1/2	1	1	3	2	4	1/2	–	1	1	1
2400	100	240	115	3/10, 3/10, 3/10, 1/10	1	2	3	2	4	1/2	2	1	3	2	3	1/2	2	1	3	3	3	1/2	–	1	1	1
2600	115	250	130	3/10, 3/10, 3/10, 1/10	1	2	3	3	3	–	2	2	3	4	4	1/2	2	1	3	3	4	1/2	–	1	1	1
3000	120	300	145	3/10, 3/10, 3/10, 1/10	1	2	4	3	4	–	2	2	4	4	4	1	2	1	4	2	5	1	–	1	1	1

Table 7.16a

APPROXIMATE CHOLESTEROL CONTENT OF SELECTED FOOD

(Values adapted from National Diet-Heart Study, 1965, and American Heart Association)

	Food Item	mgs. cholesterol per exchange
Milk	Milk, skim	8
Meat	Beef, lamb, or pork	21
	Veal	27
	Chicken	18
	Fish (steaks or fillets)	20
	Cheese, cheddar	45
	Cottage cheese, creamed	6
	Egg, whole	275
	Organ meats:	
	Liver	90
	Heart	48
	Sweetbreads	75
	Brains	2674
	Shellfish:	
	Crab or shrimp	38
	Lobster	60
	Oysters	60
Fat	Butter	20
	Vegetable Oils (corn, cottonseed, safflower, soybean)	0
	Special margarine	0
	Soft safflower margarine	0
	Mayonnaise and mayonnaise-type salad dressings	3

Table 7.16b

SUGGESTIONS FOR

Type of Hyperlipoproteinemia (Fredrickson)	MILK		VEGETABLE		FRUIT
	Allowed	Avoid	Allowed	Avoid	
TYPE I Fat: restricted to 25-35 gms/day Cholesterol: not restricted	Skim milk, buttermilk made from skim milk, dried non-fat milk	Whole milk, condensed milk, yogurt, low fat milk (1% or 2%)	Any fresh, frozen, or canned without added fat or cream sauce	Vegetables cooked with butter, margarine, meat, or cream sauce	No restrictions
TYPE II Fat: Substitute polyunsaturated fat for saturated fat* Cholesterol: intake less than 300 mgs/day	Same as above plus yogurt made from skim milk	Whole milk, condensed milk, yogurt made from whole milk	Any fresh, frozen, or canned vegetables seasoned with allowed fat.	Vegetables seasoned with fat not allowed on diet; vegetables with cream sauce	No restrictions
TYPE III Fat: Substitute polyunsaturated fat for saturated fat Cholesterol: intake less than 300 mgs/day	Same as TYPE II	Same as above	Same as above	Same as above	No restrictions
TYPE IV Fat: Substitute polyunsaturated fat for saturated fat Cholesterol: intake restricted to 300-500 mgs/day	Same as TYPE II	Same as above	Same as above	Same as above	No restrictions
TYPE V Fat: Restricted to 25-30% of total calories Substitute polyunsaturated fat for saturated fat Cholesterol: intake restricted to 300-500 mgs/day	Same as TYPE II	Same as above	Same as above	Same as above	No restrictions

Adapted from "Dietary Management of Hyperlipoproteinemia" by Donald S. Fredrickson, M.D., et al. National Heart and Lung Institute, Bethesda, Md.

Table 7.16c

HYPERLIPOPROTEINEMIA DIETS

BREAD		MEAT		FAT	
Allowed	Avoid	Allowed	Avoid	Allowed	Avoid
White, whole wheat, rye, matzo, saltines, graham crackers, cereals potatoes, all vegetables (except pork and beans)	Biscuits, corn bread, muffins, rolls, pancakes, waffles, cheese or other flavored crackers, pork & beans	Limit to 3-5 oz per day Lean, well-trimmed beef, lamb, veal, liver, chicken (without skin), fish, water-packed tuna and salmon, egg white (limit yolks to 3/week), dry cottage cheese, shellfish	Pork, fried meat, lunch meat, wieners. corned beef, fish canned in oil, goose, duck, regular ground beef, meats with sauces or gravies, cheese, peanut butter, poultry skin, spareribs, pig feet, pig tails	NONE (Medium chain triglyceride is allowed only on advice of physician)	ALL fats, avocado
Same as above	Same as above	Limit to 9 oz./day. Limit beef, lamb, pork, and ham to a 3 oz. serving only 3 x week. Chicken, turkey, veal, fish, egg white (no yolks allowed), peanut butter, dry cottage cheese	Egg yolk, wieners, lunch meats, shellfish, goose, duck, liver, heart, brains, fat meat, regular ground beef, corned beef, meats with sauces or gravies, cheese, fried meats unless fried with allowed oil, poultry skin, spareribs, pig feet, pig tails.	Safflower oil, corn oil, special margarine (liquid safflower or corn oil should be first listed ingredient on label), olives, peanuts, commercial mayonnaise *1 teaspoon of polyunsaturated fat should be consumed for each ounce of cooked meat. If more than 9 oz. of beef, lamb, pork, or ham are eaten per week, 2 teaspoons of polyunsaturated fat should be consumed for each ounce of cooked meat.	Butter, lard, bacon and drippings, sausage, hydrogenated margarine, and shortening, coconut oil and all other oils not listed, salt pork, gravies and sauces unless made with allowed fat and milk, cream cheese, cream, cracklins
Same as above	Same as above	Lean, well-trimmed beef, lamb, veal, chicken, turkey, pork, fish, creamed cottage cheese, peanut butter, egg white (no yolks allowed), low fat cheese	Egg yolk, fat meat, canned meat mixtures, duck, goose, fried meats, brains, liver, sweetbreads, shellfish, regular ground beef, lunch meats, wieners, bologna, meats with sauces or gravies, cheese (except that allowed), poultry skin, spareribs, pig feet, pig tails	Any vegetable oil (except coconut oil), special margarine (made from allowed oil with liquid oil listed as first ingredient on label), commercial mayonnaise or salad dressings containing no sour cream or cheese, avocado, nuts, olives	Butter, lard, bacon and drippings, sausage, hydrogenated shortening and margarine, coconut oil, salt pork, gravies and sauces unless made with allowed fat and skim milk, cream cheese, cream
Same as above	Same as above	Same as TYPE III with these exceptions: 3 egg yolks allowed/week OR substitute for 1 egg yolk 2 oz. cheddar cheese (limited to 2 oz. cheese/week) OR 2 oz. shellfish OR 2 oz. liver, heart, or sweetbreads	Same as TYPE III	Same as TYPE III plus commercial cheese dressings (these must be counted as cheese allowance for week)	Same as TYPE III
Same as above	Same as above	Same as TYPE III with these exceptions: 3 egg yolks allowed/week OR substitute for 1 egg yolk, 2 oz. shellfish OR 2 oz. liver, sweetbreads, or heart	Same as TYPE III	Same as TYPE III	Same as TYPE III

REFERENCES

1. The University Group Diabetes Program: A study of the
    effects of hypoglycemic agents on vascular complications
    in patients with adult-onset diabetes. Diabetes 19
    (supple. 2):747, 1970

2. The University Group Diabetes Program: Effects of hypo-
    glycemic agents on vascular complications in patients
    with adult-onset diabetes. IV. A preliminary report
    on Phenformin results. JAMA 217:777, 1971

DIET MANUALS FOR PATIENT EDUCATION

1. Davidson JK, Goldsmith MP: Diabetes Guidebook: Diet
    Section. Second edition. Emory University School of
    Medicine, 69 Butler Street, SE, Atlanta, Georgia 30303.
    Price: About $10.00

2. Meal Planning with Exchange Lists. American Diabetes
    Association, Inc., 18 East 48th Street, New York, New
    York 10017. Price: Less than $1.00

3. Schmitt G: Diabetes for Diabetics. Fourth edition.
    Diabetes Press of America, Inc., 30 S.E. 8th Street,
    Miami, Florida 33131. Price: About $10.00

4. Select-a-Meal. Diabetes Project of the North Carolina
    Regional Medical Program, Post Office Drawer 389,
    Chapel Hill, North Carolina 27514. Price: About $3.00

CHAPTER 8

Testing and the Laboratory

RALPH E. YODAIKEN, JOHN R. BORING, III
and KENNETH B. ROBERTS

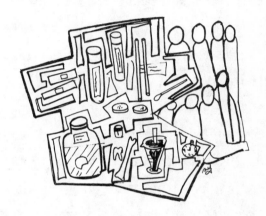

THE THREE CARDINAL questions that must be asked before taking sputum, blood, urine, or tissue from a patient or scheduling an EKG, EEG, or x-ray or any other laboratory test are:

(1) Will it provide relevant information?

(2) Is the lab competent?

(3) What will it cost the patient?

Ordering the key tests for a clinical diagnosis is a sign of competence.[8] Ordering a battery of tests for the sake of "completeness" is unnecessary and may be confusing unless

193

this is cheaper and part of multiphasic screening in which
case any positive results <u>must</u> be confirmed by specific tests
later. Even with automation, lab results are not always
accurate and the "normal" level for one lab or at one hospita
may differ significantly from the "normal" for another lab.
When dealing with an unfamiliar lab, it is sometimes worthwhile to find out about dependability and if results compare
with similar tests carried out elsewhere. The patient's
future therapy will depend on the interpretation of a normal
or abnormal result so unless the lab is well known, a surprising or unexpected figure should be checked out.

Before performing the test, even if it is only drawing
blood, the patient should be told what the test is all about
and why it is being carried out. It should not be assumed
that the patient, however young or old, is incapable of comprehension. The confidence displayed by the doctor in the
patient's ability to understand and cooperate will go a long
way to establishing good rapport between doctor and patient.
A child who has been physically or psychologically hurt by
an insensitive physician may remember the incident for life.
Patients who have had tests most frequently complain of
(1) pain, (2) careless and incompetent staff and (3) long
waiting periods. The tourniquet must be comfortable, the
needle sharp and of the smallest possible caliber (#21 will
not cause hemolysis), and above all, the patient prepared.

It is frustrating to take blood for a glucose tolerance test and then find that the patient has not been told to fast for eight hours or has not been on an adequate carbohydrate diet for three days before the test. The specimen must get to the lab in good time. Hemolysis due to dirty tubes, pulling the blood or ejecting it too rapidly is certain to produce false results, especially for potassium. Urine must be looked at in the fresh state for some tests, otherwise it is unstable, for example, for microscopy. Where relevant, the patient must be taught a technique in order to get valid results, e.g. taking a clean-catch urine specimen. The specimen must be immediately and correctly labeled. Costly errors occur because the specimens are lost or incorrectly labeled. There is nothing more chilling than losing a lymph node in transit or having a positive VDRL in a virgin because the specimen was carelessly labeled. Finally, beware of false positives or negatives, e.g. smallpox innoculation can cause a false positive VDRL, and this may even legally prevent a marriage from taking place let alone destroy the couple's trust in each other.

Physicians should also be aware that certain laboratory tests can be performed in the office with a savings in cost and time to the patient.[5]

SPECIAL TESTS

THROAT SWAB

Rheumatic fever and glomerular nephritis are theoreti-
cally preventable diseases. Streptoccal infections occur
in families.[6] In a child with a sore throat and fever the
presence of an exudate would necessitate a throat swab to
exclude group A streptococci. Streptococcal throat infections can be confirmed with a simple procedure using a commercially available sterile filter paper strip termed "Cul-
Pak". The throat swab is taken as usual and the swab is then
rubbed over the surface of the filter strip. The "Cul-Pak"
strip can then be mailed to the appropriate laboratory or
the strip, after drying, can be placed on the surface of a
commercially available blood agar plate for culture. The
streptococci grow out almost in pure culture since they are
resistant to drying while other throat organisms are not.
Further identification can be made simply by placing on the
plate before incubation an "A" disk containing bacitracin.
There will be a zone of inhibition of growth around the "A"
disk if the organism is a group A streptococcus.

CULTURE OF VAGINAL SECRETIONS

Candida albicans (moniliasis) is the most common cause
of vulvovaginitis. This occurs more frequently during pregnancy and especially in patients with diabetes. An accurate
diagnosis can be made if the vaginal secretions are cultured

on selective media such as Nickerson's Medium (Ortho); Squibb
Candida test: or Clinicult Monilia Medium (SKF). Remember,
isolation of a few colonies may not be significant. Examination of a KOH smear for the presence of pseudohyphae or
mycelia although more time consuming is still the most accurate diagnostic test. Trichomonas can be detected by direct
microscopic examination of the wet vaginal smear. Gonococcal
infection can be determined by the culture of secretions on
a selective medium such as Thayer-Martin described below.

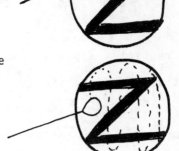

1.   Roll swab on TM medium
      in a "Z" pattern

2.   Cross streak with a sterile
      wire loop and then put the
      plate in a candle jar and
      incubate.

URINE CULTURE

Urine specimens may also be cultured in the laboratory.
A mid-stream clean-catch urine is plated on the surface of
a blood plate using a commercially available calibrated loop
which delivers 0.001 ml. of urine. If over 100 colonies
appear on the plate after incubation, this is indicative of

a urinary tract infection (100,000 bacteria per ml.). This
procedure can easily be carried out in the office.

SCREENING

With more automated methods of testing, attention must
be paid to the specificity and sensitivity of the tests used.
The more sensitive the test the higher the detection of the
disease that is allegedly measured by the marker. If a test
is too sensitive, many false positives will be obtained.
Many of the "markers" we measure are only indicators and the
patient must be treated, not the abnormal test result.[4]

THE BIOPSY

A biopsy may be painful or may bleed excessively depending upon the site and type of lesion. The patient is
frequently apprehensive regardless of the pain. Therefore,
this procedure should not be performed unless it is clearly
indicated. On the other hand some diagnoses, particularly
of tumors, cannot be made without histological confirmation.
The decision is up to the physician and good clinical judgment is needed in making that decision. If it is necessary
to excise a lesion for any other reason (a nevus for cosmetic
reasons) it should routinely be submitted for histopatholo-
gical diagnosis unless there is some valid objection (costs;
lab not available).

If a biopsy is to be of any value:

1.   The specimen must be representative.

2.   The tissue must be well fixed.

3.   A clinical history must accompany the specimen.

Scrapings from the lesion and adjacent tissue are inadequate. Some lesions are difficult enough to interpret
(for example, lymphoid tissue) when an adequate specimen is
at hand and the problem is only compounded by submitting distorted scraps of tissue. In addition to this, the form of
therapy may be dependent on complete representation of the
lesion so the tissue submitted must be large enough to clearly
show the histology of the lesion and its relationship to
surrounding tissue.

Particularly when a tumor is involved, the margin is
essential to determine if the tumor is benign or invasive
and malignant. For skin lesions it is advisable to take the
entire lesion if possible and a small rim of tissue surrounding the margin as well, providing deformity does not
result. If the lesion is too large (greater than 2 cm.) to
excise without producing a deformity, then it may be necessary to carry out an incisional biopsy in the operating room
and the tissue submitted to frozen section. If frozen sections are not possible and a tumor is involved, then the
urgency of the diagnosis should be stressed and the pathologist asked to call in the diagnosis before sending out a

formal typed note. There is some argument as to whether a
nevus should ever be incised because of the danger of making
a benign lesion malignant by traumatizing it. The patient
should always be given the benefit of the doubt. If in
doubt - DON'T!

In some instances the tissue is bound to be small, for
example in endoscopic specimens of cervical tissue. In this
case, precautions need to be taken to ensure that the area
involved in the pathological change is represented and
enough tissue is available to make a diagnosis. All too fre
quently the patient has to be recalled for a repeat biopsy
and precautions should be taken to avoid this.

Needle or aspiration biopsies have a role in very specific instances - where technically it is convenient to
needle biopsy internal organs such as the liver and the kidneys. In these two instances a needle biopsy is usually
adequate for diagnosis. Lung and bone are sometimes also
suitable but in these cases and in others, because the
specimen is small and bound to be distorted the technique
has its limitations. It is wise to consult the pathologist
prior to taking the biopsy to make sure that someone in
the lab is familiar with needle biopsies. If there is
an option between a needle biopsy and an open biopsy, then
the latter should be taken. In the case of lymphoid
tissue it is far better to remove the lymph node in an

operating room rather than to submit an aspiration biopsy.

FIXATION

Routine Sections

The key to fixation is that there should be sufficient fixative in the bottle and the tissue should be placed in the fixative as soon as possible. The biopsy material should never be left lying around on gauze nor should it be kept in an empty bottle. For most purposes 10% buffered formalin is the fixative of choice but in some cases it is not. If there is doubt about the use of formalin then again the pathologist should be consulted prior to the biopsy because later is too late. Chromaffin tissue for example, should not be fixed in formalin because this fixative may prevent the chromaffin reaction and it may be impossible for instance to differentiate histologically between a pheochromocytoma and an adrenal cortical carcinoma unless a chromaffin reaction can be done.

Electron Microscopy

Nowadays it is usual to take a specimen for electron microscopy if possible as an adjunct to diagnosis and treatment (particularly in cases of renal biopsies) or for research purposes. Formalin is not a suitable fixative for electron microscopy and the pathology laboratory should be asked to supply glutaraldehyde. Because small fragments of tissue are essential to proper fixation for electron microscopy the

tissue should be cut up with a sharp blade immediately. Thi
is best accomplished by putting a drop of previously refrigerated fixative on a sheet of dental wax, cutting the specimen up in the fixative and then pouring it into a bottle.
For renal biopsies the question of the amount of tissue
available is an important one. The operator should take
care to note how the tissue lies in the biopsy needle so
that the cortical area can be orientated. (If the orientation is lost, and only one specimen can be taken, and electron microscopy is thought to be essential to the diagnosis,
then fix the entire specimen in glutaraldehyde). A very
small snip - about one-fifth of an average specimen - is cut
off the cortical region and slipped into the glutaraldehyde
vial without further cutting. The remainder of the specimen
is put into the formaldehyde bottle or vial. The question
of taking 2 biopsies - one for routine microscopy and one fo
electron microscopy requires careful consideration and each
case must be judged on its merits. One must bear in mind
that the diagnosis is usually made on light microscopy and
the biopsy material should not be compromised. On the other
hand, if there is a greater chance of bleeding, or the patient is likely to have too few glomeruli left in any case,
then the patient should never be compromised. As a rule of
thumb - one good specimen should be enough. The tissue for
E.M. is fixed in cold glutaraldehyde and kept in a

refrigerator at 4° C for at least two hours. Many patholo-
gists do not like to read routine sections from tissue that
has been fixed in glutaraldehyde so that for routine diagnosis the remainder of the tissue should be fixed in formalin. Processing from this point on should be carried out
by the lab to which the tissue is to be submitted.

In summary: Make sure the fixative is the one required
for the diagnosis and secondly place it in the fixative immediately.

Frozen Sections

A diagnosis can usually be made on frozen section. The
reason for requiring a frozen section is to determine whether
a lesion is benign, malignant or inflammatory in order to be
able to proceed surgically while the patient is in the operating room. However, on occasion the pathologist cannot be
certain as to whether the criteria required for diagnosis
are present or not and he needs time for a formalin fixed
section. He may also require multiple sections from a single
block of tissue. Under these circumstances there is no point
in hastening the diagnosis, inconvenient as it may be to
hold up the operative procedure and return the patient to
the ward. Every pathologist of experience has seen hysterec-
tomies, mastectomies, and other operative procedures which
turned out to be entirely unnecessary carried out because
the surgeon was hasty or felt that a diagnosis could be made

on the gross specimen. If a frozen section is to be carried out then the operator should have sufficient trust in the judgment of the pathologist before asking for the biopsy to be read.

CLINICAL HISTORY

A clinical history must accompany the specimen. A renal biopsy from a patient with diabetic glomerulosclerosis may be read as a membranous glomerulonephritis if the pathologist is not aware of the abnormal glucose tolerance test. A nodular fasciitis may be diagnosed as an infiltrating fibrosarcoma if a clinical history and an accurate description of the size, color and site of the lesion are not mentioned. A well differentiated thyroid carcinoma may be read as a benign adenoma if the surgeon does not mention the attachment to underlying tissue and that area is not included in the biopsy specimen.

The history accompanying the specimen needs to be brief and should give the following details:

1.   Full name and chart number or case number

2.   Age; sex; occupation

3.   Size; color; texture of the lesion

4.   Relation to surrounding organs - fixed; infiltrating - easily shelled out

5.   Previous treatment: radiotherapy, surgery, etc.

6. Family history, if any, e.g. intestinal polyps in
    other members of the family

7. Relative investigations: Calcium, alkaline phos-
    phatase, etc.

8. Clinical diagnosis

TUBERCULIN TESTING*

The tuberculin test is an instrument for detecting infection with <u>Mycobacterium tuberculosis</u> and may be used both
as a screening instrument and as a diagnostic tool.

TUBERCULIN

Tuberculin is a biological extract of the tubercle
bacillus and is available in two forms: Purified Protein
Derivative (PPD), the refined material used as the standard
for diagnostic testing; and Old Tuberculin (OT), a more
crude product which is still used in some screening tests.

AVAILABLE PRODUCTS AND ADMINISTRATION TECHNIQUES

Although many products are commercially available, two
are by far the most popular in this country and serve as
prototypes for the others.

<u>The Tine Test</u> (Lederle): This test is of the "multiple
puncture" type and consists of a plastic body with four
"tines" or prongs coated with old tuberculin. The tines are
pressed into the skin with sufficient pressure to leave an
impression of the plastic disk which holds the tines. The

*Section written by Kenneth B. Roberts, M.D.

test is more expensive than Mantoux, but it is less demanding
since needles and syringes are not required. The greatest
drawback is that the dose of tuberculin administered is not
standardized and usually exceeds the equivalent of 5TU; this
results in difficulty in interpretation, and makes the Tine
Test an acceptable test for screening purposes only.

The Mantoux Test: The diagnostic standard is the intracu-
taneous injection of tuberculin by needle and syringe, the
Mantoux method. PPD is the product of choice and 5 Tuberculin Units (TU), the amount in 0.1 ml of PPD Standard, the
appropriate dose. Many studies, utilizing thousands of subjects, have demonstrated the validity, reliability and sensitivity of this combination of factors: 5TU dose, PPD
tuberculin and Mantoux method.

While the volar aspect of the forearm is usually selected
for testing, other convenient sites may be used if the fore-
arms are not available (because of casts or dermatological
reasons, for example).

READING AND RECORDING

Tuberculin tests are read 48-72 hours after administration.

Tine Test: The diameter of induration at the site of administration is measured and recorded in millimeters; vesiculation, if present, should be noted.

Mantoux Test: The transverse diameter of induration is

measured in millimeters and the size (NOT an interpretation such as POSITIVE or NEGATIVE) is recorded.

Erythema may be prominent but is of no significance and need not be recorded.

INTERPRETATION

Tine Test: Positive - vesiculation. (Need not be con-
               firmed with Mantoux).

               Doubtful - 2 mm or more of induration (Repeat
               with Mantoux).

               Negative - less than 2 mm of induration.

Mantoux Test: Positive - 10 mm or more of induration.

               Doubtful - 5-9 mm of induration (Retest with
               5 TU indicated).

               Negative - less than 5 mm of induration.

FALSE REACTIONS

Because the tuberculin test is an in vivo biological test, false reactions must be anticipated. Knowledge of the situations in which these responses are most likely to occur maximizes the usefulness of the test.

False Positives: While tuberculin does not elicit hypersen-sitivity reactions in persons infected with fungi, it will elicit responses from individuals infected with "atypical mycobacteria" as well as those infected with M. tuberculosis. Although the cross-reactions to atypicals tend to be smaller than reactions to M. tuberculosis, it may be difficult to discriminate the two in a given individual. For this reason,

the 5-9 mm of induration range is classified as "Doubtful";
a retest with 5TU is indicated. Using doses of tuberculin
stronger than 5TU, such as in the Tine Test or Second Strengt
(250TU) Tuberculin, will evoke more false positives and since
standards do not exist for valid interpretation of these
tests, confirmation with 5TU is necessary.

False Negatives: Whenever a tuberculin test is negative but
the clinical circumstances suggest the possibility of tuberculosis, the test should be repeated with careful attention
to details such as the tuberculin, the dose delivered intra-
cutaneously and the reading.

There will remain groups of patients who will not react
to tuberculin: those with compromised delayed hypersensitivity responses due to disease (such as Hodgkins or Sarcoidosis) or to medication (such as steroids or immunosup-
presives); those with overwhelming illness, those with
measles or who have recently received live viral vaccines;
those infected with M. tuberculosis too recently to have
become tuberculin-positive; and those whose sensitivity to
tuberculin has waned with advancing age. While a second
test with 5TU is indicated for all these groups, it is particularly noteworthy in the aged, where a "booster effect"
seems to recall reactivity to tuberculin.[3] (Repeat skin
testing does not cause sensitivity in uninfected individuals)

The percentage of false negative responses accumulated will depend in large part on the prevalence of the clinical conditions enumerated above in the population being tested. False negative reactions which cannot be accounted for occur in less than one-half of one percent of patients.[7]

REFERENCES

1.   American Thoracic Society Committee on Diagnostic Skin
      Testing: The tuberculin skin test.   Amer Rev Resp Dis
      104:769, 1971

2.   Edwards PQ, Edwards LB: Story of the tuberculin test
      from an epidemiologic viewpoint.   Amer Rev Resp Dis
      81:1, 1960

3.   Ferebee S, Mount F: Evidence of booster effect in
      serial tuberculin testing.   Amer Rev Resp Dis 88:118,
      1963

4.   Fiumara NJ: A laboratory test is not a diagnosis.
      JAMA 217:71, 1971

5.   Griner PF, Liptzin B: Use of the laboratory in a
      teaching hospital: Implications for patient care, edu-
      cation and hospital costs.   Ann Int Med 75:157, 1971

6.   Haggerty RJ, Meyer RJ: Streptococcal infections in
      families - factors altering individual susceptibility.
      Pediatrics 29:539, 1962

7.   Kent DC, Schwartz R: Active pulmonary tuberculosis
      with negative tuberculin skin reactions.   Amer Rev Resp
      Dis 95:411, 1967

8.   Laboratory tests: Misuse and abuse.   JAMA 218:90, 1971
      (Editorial)

Cancer Screening
–Some Aspects

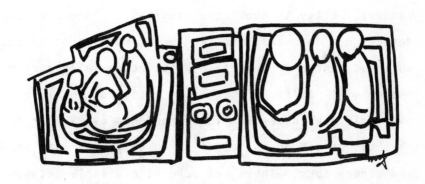

THERE HAS BEEN a steady slow rise in the incidence
of cancer. There were 650,000 cases in 1972 with
an annual death rate of 345,000 Americans estimated to increase to 510,000 deaths in the year 2000.[4] This increase
is real and is due to an increased life expectancy and awareness of the nature of the disease both among physicians and
patients.

Once cancer is diagnosed it has a devastating effect
on the patient, the family, and the physician. It requires
a complete reorganization of family structure, preparation
for the possible impending death, and carries with it an awe-
some emotional and economic burden. Therefore, the physician
should be as certain as is possible within scienfitic limits

211

before making a firm diagnosis. Cancer diagnosis and its treatment require a multi-disciplinary approach involving the physician, pathologist, cytopathologist, radiologist, radio therapist, surgeon and social worker.

At this time since we do not know the etiology of most cancers, we try to abort the progress of tumors by early detection. This has resulted in an improvement in the prognosis of cancer from certain sites, especially carcimona of the cervix. At the present time it is not possible for every citizen in the USA to be screened every year for cancer The best we can do is select the high cancer risk population and screen them. There are several available methods, principally exfoliative cytology, x-ray, and blood tests. The first of these methods, although described by Papanicolaou as early as 1928 was largely ignored. The practicality of his finding was not realized until the publication in 1943 of his classic monograph with Traut, "Diagnosis of Uterine Cancer by the Vaginal Smear".[3] Since that time, the "Pap" smear has become a routine screening technique for cervical and uterine cancer. Now it is also applied to the detection of pulmonary, oral, breast, GI and GU cancers as well. Further it is used for diagnosing the nature of pleural, pericardial and abdominal effusions, breast secretions, lymph node and cystic or solid tumor aspirate.

Application of this technique makes three major demands on the physician. First, as stated in the description of the method, the limitations as well as the benefits of the technique must be clearly understood. A close relationship should exist between the clinician and cytopathologist. Secondly the practice of taking the specimen must be exact. Although it is a relatively inexpensive procedure, it is time consuming. Thirdly the patient must be informed of the significance of the test and reassured if necessary.[1]

Since exfoliative cytology (cytopathology) is the best method of detecting some cancers, particularly cancer of the cervix, and since the diagnosis may depend on the accuracy of the technique, it is dealt with in detail in the following chapter.

CHAPTER 9

Exfoliative Cytopathology

ZUHER NAIB

THE BODY TISSUES, because of the need for contin-
uous renewal, desquamate cells in an unceasing
manner. Some of these cells accumulate in natural cavities
and recesses and others are lost from the surface or through
the gastro-intestinal tract. Exfoliative cytopathology is
the study of the morphology of these spontaneously or artificially exfoliated cells to detect and diagnose various
diseases and neoplasia of different organs.[2]

ADVANTAGES

1. The method does not produce any injury to the tissues
    and allows frequent repetition of cellular sampling.
    (Important in the evaluation of the progression or
    post-treatment regression of a lesion).
2. It diagnoses the pathology of a large area, with the
    cells originating from a wider surface than those seen
    in a biopsy.

3. Cellular samples often originate from areas inaccessible
    to a biopsy (bottom of a diverticulum, crypt, gland,
    etc.).

4. Some diseases are easier to diagnose with a smear than
    a section. (Example: genital herpesvirus or tricho-
    monos infection, etc.).

5. The method is rapid, simple (no microtome or paraffin
    embedding is needed) and cheap (average cost is five
    dollars).

LIMITATIONS

1. The screening of a smear can be time-consuming.

2. The interrelation of the cells cannot be determined.
    Neighboring cells in a smear often originate from dis-
    tant points.

3. The relation of the cells to the stroma cannot be es-
    tablished. (Important for example in the differentia-
    tion of an invasive carcinoma fron one in situ).

4. The size and stage of a lesion cannot be determined by
    the study of exfoliated cells. The number of diagnos-
    tic cells in a smear has no relation to the size of the
    lesion. For example, a cervical in situ cancer will
    have more diagnostic cells in a vaginal smear than a
    large fungating, invasive one.

5. Sample of the cells studied may originate from an un-
    wanted site (for example, rectal cells in a vaginal

smear, liver cells in an ascitic fluid, etc).

VAGINAL CYTOLOGY

In gynecology and obstetrics, cytology has three major applications:

1.   Detection and diagnosis of cervical, endocervical, endometrial and ovarian cancerous and precancerous lesions.

2.   Assessment of endocrine functions by examination of the vaginal cells.

3.   Diagnosis of the presence and nature of genital infections.

COMBINED VAGINAL SMEAR

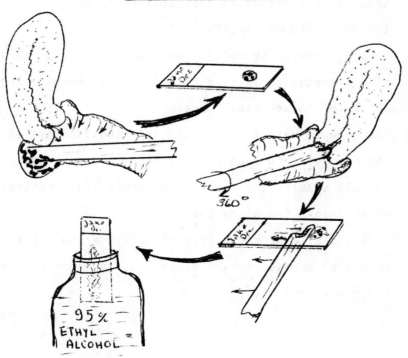

TECHNIQUE

1. Identify slide by writing name of the patient on the frosted end and complete requisition by indicating date of last menstrual period (LMP) and the previous menstrual period (PMP), age of the patient, known pregnancy and gynecologic symptoms.

2. Remove all talcum powder from gloves before touching the patient, instruments or slides.

3. Several droplets of vaginal pool secretion and endocervical aspiration are removed from the posterior fornix and endocervical os.

4. Droplets are placed on the labelled slide one inch from the end. (DO NOT SMEAR).

5. Obtain cervical scraping from the squamo-columnar junction by rotating spatula 360° around external os, high up in the endocervical canal.

6. The scraped material is mixed with the droplets of vaginal pool and endocervical mucus and smeared by quickly drawing the spatula or finger from combined drops across the slide twice.

7. IMMEDIATELY drop slide into 95% ethyl alcohol fixative or use an aerosol spray (water soluble commercial hair spray will do).

CYTOLOGIC REPORTING IN CANCER SCREENING

The numberical classification (Class I to Class V) used in the past is not acceptable. This "number game" often hides the ignorance of the cytopathologist and may result in the misinterpretation of the report by the clinician. A simplified descriptive system and a diagnosis should be rendered similar to the one given in surgical pathology. A recommendation based on the morphology of the cells should be included to assist the clinician in the handling of the patient. If this is not done, the clinician should ask for clarification.

APPLICATION

The universal use of the routine genital scraping, "Pap" test, in all women above the age of 16 may well eliminate cervical cancer as a cause of death. Invasive epidermoid cervical cancer develops from an early asymptomatic lesion limited to the cervical epithelium (carcinoma in situ) which is readily and effectively (95%) detectable by cytology. This early discovery and prompt therapy produces a 100% cure. In invasive, symptomatic advanced cancer, cytology is useful only to evaluate the result of the treatment and to differentiate, for example, radiation changes from a persisting or recurrent carcinoma. A biopsy should be taken of ALL grossly visible suspicious cervical lesions. Negative cytological findings DO NOT rule out a neoplasm. If there is any

evidence that a lesion exists, the smear should be repeated
and other detection means should be used. Pregnancy is not
a contraindication for taking a smear. The detection rate
for cancer does not change.

Endometrial and ovarian adenocarcinoma in 60% of the
cases spontaneously exfoliate neoplastic cells to the vagina
and can be readily recognized in a vaginal pool smear. The
detection rate approaches 90% when endometrial irrigation,
lavage or brush method is used.

The detection and treatment of an early adenocarcinoma
will save the life of the majority of patients.

ASSESSMENT OF INFLAMMATORY CONDITIONS

The two most common symptoms of genital inflammation,
pruritis (itching) and leukorrhea (vaginal discharge) are
the most frequent reasons for women to seek medical advice.

The examination of a smear will readily differentiate
and diagnose the following inflammatory conditions by the
recognition of the organisms involved or the cellular changes
it produces.

1.   Bacterial (Doderlein's bacillus, gonococcus, tubercu-
     losis, various cocci infections.

2.   Protozoal (trichomonas, entamoeba histolytica, schisto-
     somia infection)

3.   Fungal (monilia)

4. Viral (herpes, TRIC agent, adenovirus, cytomegalic
    inclusion disease)
5. Hormonal (atrophic vaginitis

NON-GENITAL CYTOLOGY

LUNG

Early detection of bronchogenic cancer is the only hope for cure. The rapid increase of the incidence of lung cancer (18 times as high for men as it was 40 years ago) makes the use of cytology, as one of several detection procedures, even more urgent and important.

Because of the cost, low yield and difficulty in processing the specimens, pulmonary cytology is not yet used as a screening method for lung diseases of the healthy general population as is the case for genital cancer. It is mainly used to detect and determine the nature of the pulmonary neoplasm from symptomatic patients (hemoptisis) or from those with a silent but suspicious pulmonary lesion as seen in chest x-ray. Exception is the use of pulmonary cytological screening of high-risk groups of men with a history of heavy cigarette smoking of several years' duration or long exposure to polluted air (certain mining and chemical industries workers for example). Approximately 90% of all pulmonary neoplasms can be detected and typed by examination of the cells in a sputum and bronchial washing.

NOTE: ONE SPUTUM SERIES consists of FIVE DAILY, FRESH SPE-
CIMENS (Pick-up of primary bronchogenic carcinoma is thus
increased from 60% in one sputum to over 90% in a series.
DO NOT submit 24 hour specimens.)
Other techniques used include aerosal inhalation for patients
with slight or no expectoration; bronchial, tracheo-bronchial
aspiration and bronchial washings.
BODY CAVITY FLUIDS

The presence of effusions in a body cavity is always
abnormal. The transudates are the result of physio-chemical
alteration of the body fluid (increased venous pressure or
decreased osmotic pressure). Low in protein and specific
gravity, they are clear or yellowish with little tendency
to clot and contain only a few small mesothelial cells, his-
tiocytes and inflammatory cells.

The exudates result from the irritation of the serous
mucosa by such agents as cancer, inflammation, foreign body,
hemorrhage, etc. They have a high protein content and specific gravity and may contain large reactive mesothelial
cells, abundant inflammatory cells and cancer cells. Exfoliative cytology is used not only to detect the involvement
of the serosa with a neoplasm (mainly metastatic in type)
but also to determine the nature and cause of the effusion
by the analysis of the nature and abundance of its non-
neoplastic cellular components (type of inflammatory

cells, viral changes, presence of microorganisms, etc.).

MISCELLANEOUS SPECIMENS

Gastro-Intestinal Tract

The scraping of oral lesions will produce cells with morphological changes diagnostic of various viral (herpes, measles, chicken pox) fungal (monilia) and other inflammation (lichen, planus, pemphigus, stomatitis, radiation and Carrier-White's disease). The early buccal mucosa cancer often looks grossly like a small red, innocuous benign irritation spot which, if scraped, will provide easily recognized tumor cells. The washing or brush scraping of the esophageal and gastric mucosa exfoliate cells is diagnostic of various malignant and non-malignant lesions with a high rate of accuracy. It is important to obtain the specimen only after cleaning the gastric-esophageal mucosa from food particles, mucous and cellular debris.

The nature of a suspected colonic lesion can be diagnosed by the examination of the exfoliated cells found in the last enema washing when the fluid return is almost clear. The detection rate of colonic cancer varies depending on the location, size and nature of the lesion and the cytologic method used.

Urinary Tract

The urine, preferably catheterized, obtained from the bladder, ureter or pelvis may contain, besides the normal transitional cells, inflammatory and neoplastic cells, variou

casts and crystals. Their correct interpretation helps in

the clinical management of the patient with urinary symptoms.

Prostate and Seminal Vesicles

The rectal massage of these organs produces a secretion

appearing at the tip of the urethral meatus which, when

smeared and examined, may detect the presence of a neoplasm

or help in the diagnosis of the nature of the inflammatory

disease.

Breast

Nipple secretion, cyst fluid and solid breast mass

needle aspiration can provide cellular evidence of the pres-

ence of various neoplastic and non-neoplastic breast diseases

It is especially useful in the diagnosis of intraductal

papillomas, infiltrating duct carcinoma and nipple superfi-

cial carcinoma or Paget's disease.

Other Sites

Spinal fluid, lymph node aspiration and needle aspira-

tion of almost any organ of the body may be useful but are

not the primary methods of diagnosis. Etiological methods

are important when a tissue biopsy is not indicated, too

dangerous or impossible. Scraping of the various skin and

eye lesions may also provide the rapid specific diagnosis

often needed for a successful treatment.

REFERENCES

1. Kegeles SS: Attitudes and behavior of the public re-
    garding cervical cytology: Current findings and new
    directions for research. J Chronic Dis 20:199, 1967

2. Naib Z: Exfoliative Cytopathology. Boston, Little
    Brown & Co., 1970

3. Papanicoloau GN, Traut HF: Diagnosis of Uterine Car-
    cinoma by the Vaginal Smear. New York, Commonweath
    Fund, 1943

4. Silverberg E, Holleb AI: Cancer statistics 1972. A
    Cancer Journal for Clinician 22:1, 1972

CHAPTER 10

Measuring

NAOMI BAUMSLAG, EDWARD B. SILBERSTEIN
and MARTIN SAIDLEMAN

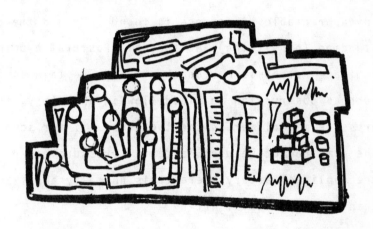

TECHNIQUES OF MEASUREMENT are constantly changing.

Individual variations, defective instruments and errors in usage or interpretation can influence values. Results should be standardized and compared in similar groups. Check to see if values obtained vary according to the time of day and keep flow charts.

In the 1800's the thermometer was used solely by the physician. Nowadays many housewives can use a thermometer. This may happen to the sphygmomanometer as more sophisticated techniques for measurement of blood pressure are developed.

227

BLOOD PRESSURE

"Blood pressure" refers to the systemic arterial blood pressure. Blood pressure varies in vessels of different caliber. Unless stated otherwise, the pressure in the brachial artery is always measured. Readings should be taken on both arms at the first examination and subsequently, if any appreciable difference is found. Record the pressure standing (or sitting) and supine. Postural hypotension may indicate autonomic neuropathy. Under certain circumstances, such as obstruction to blood flow in an artery, the blood pressure may differ in the two arms. If for some reason the arms cannot be used, arterial pressure can be taken at the popliteal artery where it is normally about 20 mm. higher than in the brachial artery.

The blood pressure of any normal person is subject to considerable variation, but the systolic pressure varies more than the diastolic. Both pressures are usually higher in the upright than the recumbent position. The systolic pressure is normally lower during sleep than when awake, sometimes by as much as 25 to 30 mm. The blood pressure can rise in response to exertion, emotion, stress and pain. The diastolic pressure represents a constant load imposed upon the walls of the arterial system and more accurately reflects the degree of peripheral resistance.

Obliterate the pulse fully, inflating the cuff to approximately 150 to 200 mm. Air is then gradually released,
and a series of tapping sounds will be heard with the ste-
thoscope, giving the rhythm of the heart beat as blood flow
increases in the artery under the cuff. The point at which
these sounds are first heard indicates the systolic blood
pressure. This is the upper of the two points recorded as
the blood pressure. As the pressure in the sphygmomanometer
is gradually reduced by releasing air, the sounds first
audible at the level of systolic pressure will become louder
and, although changing somewhat in character, remain fairly
constant until the point is reached generally 20 mm. or
more below the systolic reading. Here the relatively sharp
tapping sounds change into dull, feeble thuds; the reading
at this point of change represents the diastolic pressure.
At this point, the sounds generally disappear. A blood
pressure reading of 120/80 means that the systolic pressure
is 120 mm. Hg. and diastolic 80 mm. Hg. In fat patients it
is frequently difficult to pick up the changing sounds.
Watch the needle or the mercury of the manometer. It will
move with the pulse beat as the sounds become audible.

In normal healthy adults, the range of systolic blood
pressure is 90 to 130 mm.; or diastolic pressure 60-85 mm.
As a rule, when the systolic pressure tends to remain in
the lower range, the diastolic pressure is also low. In

children, the figures are lower than in adults, averaging
50-60 mm. systolic and 30-40 mm. diastolic at birth and
gradually increasing to adolescence when there is a sharper
rise to the adult level.

A systolic pressure over 140 mm. and a diastolic over
90 mm. persisting before middle age should be regarded as
abnormal if this level is found on three separate blood
pressure determinations on three different days. In middle
life, the upper limit of normal may be somewhat higher.

TEMPERATURE

Try to keep a record of basal temperature for the patient. The "normal" exhibits considerable variation from
patient to patient and even in the same patient at different
times of day. Sometimes a child who looks out of sorts, is
restless, irritable, and loses his appetite, has a high
temperature. Parents should be shown how to use a thermometer correctly.

RECTAL TEMPERATURE

Rectal temperature is usually taken in infants and occasionally used for uncooperative or irrational patients.
Rectal temperatures are contraindicated when surgery of the
rectum has been performed or when there is acute, severe
inflammation of the rectum. In infants, rectal temperatures
almost always may be obtained even in the presence of diarrhea; but the thermometer must be inserted gently and the

patient never left unattended.

The thermometer must first be wiped clean of sterilizing medium and shaken firmly by holding it between the thumb and forefinger until the mercury line reaches its lowest marking. Do not touch the mercury bulb or you will be recording your own temperature. Lubricate with a small amount of vaseline up to approximately one inch above the bulb to minimize irritation and facilitate the insertion of the thermometer. With the infant on his stomach or side, separate the buttocks so that the anal sphincter is clearly seen. Then insert the thermometer to a distance of about one inch. The thermometer should be held in place with one hand while the other hand has firm control of the buttocks and torso of the child. Hold in place for two to three minutes, so there is sufficient time for it to register. Then remove the thermometer and wipe it clean with a tissue, taking care not to touch the bulb, and read it. The normal rectal temperature ranges up to about 99.5° although 100° Fahrenheit may be normal in some children. Crying can raise the temperature a degree or two. After an epileptic convulsion the temperature may also rise.

ORAL TEMPERATURE

If the thermometer has been stored in a chemical solution, wipe it dry with a firm twisting motion using clean paper or clean tissue. Grasp the thermometer firmly with

the thumb and forefinger and with firm wrist movements, shake
the thermometer until the mercury line reaches the lowest
marking as noted previously for the rectal temperature. Read
the thermometer by holding it horizontally at eye level, rotating it until the line of mercury comes into view. Then
place the mercury bulb of the thermometer under the patient's
tongue and instruct him to close his lips tightly, leaving
the thermometer in place for two to three minutes. Read the
thermometer as described above and place it in the cleansing
solution.

Note that if the patient has had a hot or cold drink or
smoked a cigarette in the last fifteen minutes, the temperature will be raised and will not be a true reflection.

AXILLARY TEMPERATURE

Useful in children and adults. Usually one degree
lower than oral temperature. The thermometer must be kept
in place for 10 minutes, however.

MENTAL FUNCTION

The physician may have to decide if parents are mentally
capable of looking after themselves or rearing children; if
a child should go to a regular school; or if an adult is
capable of caring for himself. Subjective observations alone
are not enough and special tests may be needed to determine
the "measurable mental base" on which an individual functions so that a person will not be put in a position that
requires more than he can mentally perform.

There are no ideal measuring tools or tests for assessing mental function nor are there fixed units of intellectual function. Measures such as "mental age", "intelligence quotient", "percentile rank" are derived concepts relevant to performance in a particular test at a special time. However there are tests which, if considered in terms of their limitations, can be used to measure intelligence or level of mental ability.[8] Tests used must (1) be sensitive to pick up individual differences; (2) be reliable and reproducible in the same subjects under similar circumstances; and (3) test what they set out to measure. An intelligence test must correlate highly with criteria such as learning ability in school or at work. Limiting factors as to performance at a given time may be physical, emotional or even environmental, and should be ruled out if suspected. Once some of these factors are altered, a repeat test may give a different result.

Remember that any test is:

1. Manmade - and approximates a controlled experiment with standard stimuli and measurable responses evaluated against "normal data".

2. Made up of behavior samples and includes basic types of functioning such as sensimotor, sensory discrimination, attention, memory, judgment, reasoning, verbal comprehension and expression as well as abstraction or generalization.

3. Presupposes a basic minimum of opportunities for learning and development. Where there is a grossl deprived physical, emotional or cultural environment, marked sensory impairment etc. should be reevaluated when developmental impediments are corrected.

Special tests should be carried out by a clinical psychologist who is able to clarify without helping, knows how to enlist cooperation without introducing bias and may independently add to observations made.

ALERT LIST FOR ABNORMAL MENTAL FUNCTION

1. Difficult delivery
2. Family history   (Huntington's Chorea)
3. Birth defect
4. Delayed milestones
5. Intelligent parents who are defensive and make a great fuss over small achievements
6. Slow learners, slow speakers
7. Behavior problems

In some cases the problem is with the parents who may see the child as dull or slow and treat him protectively. The child may be slow in comparison to a very bright sister or brother. The fear of mental illness and its associated social stigmata can make it difficult to get at the truth easily.

Specific tests that are used:[1,2,3,4,6,11]

1. Gessell Developmental Schedule
    4-56 weeks

2. Gessell Infant Intelligence
    2 months-5 years

3. Stanford-Binet
    2 years or more

4. Wechsler Intelligence Scale for Children (WISC)
    Use in the 5-16 year old age group

5. Columbia Mental Maturity Scale
    2 1/2-16 years. This test is particularly helpful
    with children that have speech or motor difficulty
    as it requires non-verbal responses.

6. Wechsler Adult Intelligence Scale (WAIS)
    Used for adults

7. Vineland Social Maturity Scale
    This test is useful for either infants or adults
    when there is a need to assess areas such as
    (1) self help (2) locomotion (3) occupation
    (4) communication (5) self direction (6) sociali-
    zation.

When it comes to placement of children or adults in
institutions, special schools or special classes, the IQ
rating is still used for screening. An IQ of

0- 25 =	Profound Retardation	80- 89 =	Dull Normal
26- 50 =	Severe Retardation	90-109 =	Normal Average
51- 70 =	Moderate Retardation	110-119 =	Above Average
71- 79 =	Mild Retardation	120-129 =	Superior Intelligence

Although this classification is used there are degrees
of overlap. There have been several instances where the
unilateral decision of an inexperienced school psychologist
or physician turned out to be an unfortunate error of judgment. It may be quite wrong to accept an individual opinion
when the child deviates from the norm. Making a lifetime
decision for an individual requires a consensus of informed
opinions.

VISION[4,7,10]

Vision problems present a major source of correctable
pathology in the younger age groups. Between 5-10% of pre-
school children have visual impairment. This increases to
20-30% in the mid school years. Early detection is important.   Eye examinations should be carried out periodically.
INFANCY

Examination of the newborn's eyes may be hampered by
the use of $AgNo_3$ and a resultant chemical conjunctivitis.
The eyes often appear filled with mucous for 3-5 days and
an adequate examination is frequently difficult. Strabismus
should be critically evaluated if it persists beyond 3
months.

Examination

Fundiscopic: In premature infants this will allow the examiner to detect approximately 50% of blindness due to congenita
causes. A word about the technique of examining the infant's

eyes - the opthalmoscope should be held in a fixed position
while the head of the infant is simultaneously held still.
The eye movements of the infant will cross the field of the
opthalmoscope thus allowing fleeting glimpses of the fundi.

Response to Light: Check the infant's response to the direction of light by using a flashlight held in front of the eyes
and moving it slowly to one side or another.

Corneal Reflexes: Occular alignment can be estimated by
noting the corneal reflexes.

PRESCHOOL CHILD

   Success in testing the preschool child lies in patience,
adequate preparation of the child, and skill. Tests are
often misleading and must be repeated to confirm suspected
pathology.

Testing Visual Acuity

   There are many charts and devices used for testing
visual acuity. One must always remember to test each eye
separately. Unilateral amblyopia (lazy eye) may go unde-
tected and therefore untreated unless each eye is tested
separately. It is often impossible to correct unilateral
amblyopia beyond five years of age.

Snellen Test

   This test is useful in children from three to five years
of age. The most inexpensive and accurate test is the
Snellen Illiterate "E" Test. The child should practice at
a distance of one to two feet by pointing his finger in the

same direction as the fingers of the "E" (or table legs).
The test should then be performed at a distance of 20 feet,
properly illuminated with a 75 watt bulb in a gooseneck lamp
with a metal shade. The source of illumination should be
about five feet from the card. Although there is a great
deal of controversy, a visual acuity of less than 20/40 in
a three year old or 20/30 in a 4-5 year old is used as the
basis for referral. Further studies are also indicated if
there is a difference of more than one line in the visual
acuity of both eyes. Standardize referral criteria with
the physician concerned. If the patient cannot relate to
the Snellen Illiterate "E" Test, use picture cards such as
the Allen cards or toy tests such as the "Stycar" set of
tests. Repeated test failures in spite of adequate preparations should alert the examiner to investigate further.
Emotional or physical handicaps may be present.

Occular Alignment

Estimate occular alignment and coordination by rating
the corneal reflex, direct observation or a cover test. A
cover test is performed by placing a light 13-15" in front
of the eye and covering one eye. If excess lateral squint
is present, the eye will move to a pathological position
when covered and noticeable movement toward the light when
uncovered. Misalignment should be referred promptly.

External Inspection

Unexplained or prolonged irritation, inflammation or discharge should be referred to an opthalmologist. A red eye might have been simple conjunctivitis but again it might be due to a corneal ulcer, lacrimal stenosis, uveitis, or congenital glaucoma all of which may require surgical treatment.

SCHOOL AGE

Testing should be done with a standard Snellen alphabet chart or a similar device. Take care to see that the light is adequate. The child at five or six should also be given a color blind test (Hardy-Rand Rittler Test or Ishihara Test). Adequate and proper lighting is a must for reliability. During the high school years, depth perception should be tested. The Wirt steroacuity test or a comparable test may be used. An estimate of occular alignment and external inspection should always be done.

HEARING[1,5]

The early diagnosis and treatment or prevention of hearing loss is essential in minimizing problems. Children with hearing impairment are not only handicapped in the development of communication skills, but often have problems and distortions in emotional and social development.

Statistics vary, but around 4-5% of school-age children will not pass "screening" tests and about 2% of these will

actually have hearing impairments requiring medical attention.

HEARING IMPAIRMENTS

Conductive hearing loss refers to a loss when sound is
transmitted freely through the ear to the end organ.

Sensoneural refers to loss of hearing due to impairment of the sense organ and/or auditory nerve pathway.

There may be a combination of the above involving different physiologic and psychologic aspects.

TESTS

Non-Audiometric

Effective screening testing of the infant requires
sound presented without any visible clues as to its source,
and at a level of loudness easily heard but not startlingly
loud. For the infant, hearing is a reflex reaction to sound
stimuli. Response is variable with eye-blinking, gross body
reflexes, etc., and is not considered prognostic.

Audiometric

Audiometry is the process of measuring hearing levels
with an instrument which produces audible tones and can be
calibrated and controlled in both frequency and intensity.
Standards of calibration have been developed by the International Standard Organization (ISO). An audiometric evaluation with a frequency of 500, 1000, 2000, 4000, and 8000

at 25 DB (ISO), given around four years of age, will tend
to give an accurate assessment of auditory defects.
Maturation of the child is important in determining reliability, but a failure at any frequency warrants referral.

Suspected hearing impairment obviously requires careful
attention and special hearing tests in a controlled environment with little or no extraneous noise. In general,
one could follow the following criteria for instituting
referral:

ISO DB	
30-35	loss of two frequencies; 500, 1000, 2000 in either ear
40 or above	loss of one frequency; 500, 1000, 2000 in either ear
40 or above	loss of both 4000 and 8000 frequency

Children who are tested and have an ISO level of 10-26
DB are considered within normal limits and have no difficulty
with faint speech. You may compare the loudness in DB that
it takes and how much is required to overcome a loss in sensitivity for speech.

Hearing Level DB ISO tested at 500, 1000 2000 frequency	Hearing Loss	Types of Speech Child can Understand
27-40	Mild	Difficulty with faint speech
41-55	Moderate	Difficulty with normal speech
56-70	Moderately severe	Difficulty with loud speech
71-90	Severe	Only shouted or amplified speech
91 +	Profound	Cannot understand even amplified

This chart points out the critical relationship between hearing and speech.[9] Inattention, failure to respond appropriately to sound, behavior problems, and failure to develop speech and language commensurate with age are among the leading symptoms which should alert the clinician to explore hearing problems.

Choice of Audiometers is well documented,[4] but which-ever machine is used, remember that the testing environment must be relatively quiet and free from distractions in order to produce an accurate test. It is questionable whether group testing has any advantages over individual testing. Many of those tested in groups must be retested, and individual patient reactions are lost to the tester. The initial audiometric screening is often called a "sweep" test, because the operator sweeps through the selected frequencies at pre-set intensities.

Before referral is made, it is suggested that all failures be retested and a threshold hearing test performed (the least intensities heard at selected frequencies). Most of all, remember to assess the person and not the results of the test alone.

REFERENCES

1. Committee on Standards of Child Health Care: Standards
    of Child Health Care. Second edition. Evanston, Americ
    Academy of Pediatrics, 1972

2. Doll EA: Vineland Social Maturity Scale: Manual of
    Directions. Minneapolis, Minnesota, Educational Test
    Bureau Education Publishers, 1947

3. Goodenough FL: Measurement of Intelligence by Drawings.
    New York, World Book Co., 1926

4. Green M, Haggerty RJ: Ambulatory Pediatrics. Phila-
    delphia, W. B. Saunders Co., 1968

5. Harrington DA: Services for the Child Who Is Hard of
    Hearing. U.S. Dept. HEW, Children's Bureau Publication
    No. 402, 1963

6. Illingworth RS: The predictive value of development
    tests in the first year with special reference to the
    diagnosis of mental subnormality. J Child Psychol 2:
    210, 1961

7. Lin-Fu JS: Vision Screening of Children. U.S. Dept
    of HEW, MCHS, Washington, 1971

8. Lyman H: Test Scores and What They Mean. New York,
    Prentice Hall, 1962

9. Morley ME: The Development and Disorders of Speech in
    Childhood. Baltimore, Williams & Wilkins, 1962

10. Savitz RA, Reed RB, Valadian I: Vision Screening in
    the Pre-School Child. Children's Bureau Publication
    No. 414. U.S. Dept of HEW, 1964

11. Wechsler D: The Measurement and Appraisal of Adult
    Intelligence. Baltimore, Williams & Wilkins, 1958

CHAPTER 11

Environmental Pathology

RALPH E. YODAIKEN

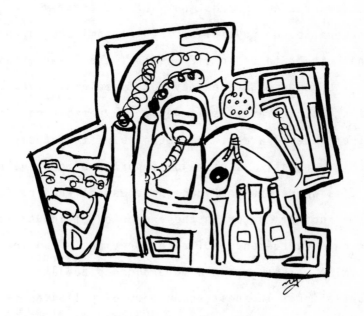

UNTIL RECENTLY ENVIRONMENTAL pathology was almost
a medical curiosity - mainly limited to infectious
and neoplastic diseases on a geographic or epidemiological
basis on the one hand and industrial or occupational diseases on the other hand. Several factors have changed this.
Population shifts, particularly following World War II, have
brought infectious diseases to areas which were previously

free of them. In part this is associated with antibiotic
therapy since resistant strains have emerged sometimes to
be carried from one country to another. Gonorrhea and malaria brought back from Vietnam to the U.S.A. are examples of
this. This means that a known disease, previously respon-
sive to a specific therapeutic agent, may present an unexpected problem in treatment, or a disease may be relatively
unknown to the physician. Schistosomiasis is not endemic in
the United States so cirrhosis of the liver or a stricture
of the colon or ureter may not immediately evoke a diagnosis
of schistosomiasis as it would in Puerto Rico, Africa or
other endemic areas. Yet because of the population shifts,
schistosomiasis is of major importance in large American
cities where Puerto Ricans have established residence.[1]

Another factor is the explosion of industrial wastes
on our environment. Diseases previously confined to factory
or mine workers are now more commonplace among the general
population. The best known form of pollution is air pollution because it produces so many obvious side effects - eye,
nose and throat irritation, headaches and sinus problems.
Asthma, emphysema and chronic bronchitis are all tied into
air pollution on a seasonal basis. Disastrous effects of
air pollution have been associated with temperature inver-
sions. The Meuse River Valley - Belgium in 1930; the disas-
ter of Donora, Pennsylvania in 1948; the fogs of London in

1952; and the New York city episodes of the early '60's are
the most frequently quoted examples of this. The factors
responsible for these lung problems are noxious gases, sul-
phur oxides, nitrogen oxides, ozone, hydrocarbons and particulates carried in the ambient air from factory sites
through the cities.

Awareness of these lung irritants is important because
physicians have to introduce a new set of possibilities into
the differential diagnosis of lung disease. Allergy in the
form of asthma may not be idiopathic or related to pollen.
It may be due to chemical contamination from industrial
plants and therefore related to temperature inversion, particularly during the summer. Careful assessment of the
clinical history, its relationship to weather and location
are relevant. Chronic bronchitis, a winter ailment, is
common in city dwellers. Smoking further complicates the
lung condition but the disease is not limited to smokers.

In addition, recent investigations have shown that berrylium and asbestos are among the particulates carried through
the city streets, invading the lungs of people not involved
in processing or manufacturing contaminating articles. Nowadays a differential diagnosis for tuberculosis is sarcoidosis,
berryliosis and asbestosis.

Personal habits, occupation, the location of the patient's residence, the type of housing and its proximity to

traffic lanes are all important to an environmental history.
Lead poisoning is a typical example. Lead poisoning is an
occupational hazard among factory workers where lead is used
(battery manufacturers). Blood lead levels are also high
among those who inhale automobile fumes continually - traffic
tunnel operators, taxi drivers, etc. Recently, it was suggested that hyperactivity in New York city children may be
related in some cases to lead blood levels lower than previously considered toxic (below 55 micrograms/100 ml. but
above 35 micrograms/100 ml.).[9] Although this needs to be
confirmed, the investigation reinforces the need to consider
the adverse effects of lead poisoning in problem children
living in polluted cities. Usually lead poisoning in children results from ingestion of lead paint from the walls of
older houses. But there are many other sources such as lead
released from ceramic table ware and ingested with food and
drink. Since lead arsenate is used as a pesticide, it may
be found in soils and on sprayed fruit and vegetables. It
also occurs in relatively high concentrations in oysters
from polluted waters.

Water and solid waste are common sources of pollution.
Water is a carrier of bacteria or viruses, mineral, chemical
and radioactive pollutants. Outbreaks of enteritis have
been tracked to polluted water, particularly in rainy seasons.
Contaminated wells are a source of family pollution, and wells

are common in rural America. It has been suggested that
naturally occurring goitrogens may be carried by water to
endemic goiter areas.[13]

Pollutant burdens carry the hazard of tetragenic, muto-
geric and carcinogenic effects. Diagnosis may be made by
blood levels or tissue biopsy, but sometimes the etiological
agents may disappear from the blood and tissues before the
pathology becomes clinically evident. For example, it may
not be possible to detect raised manganese blood levels in
neurological disorders produced by manganese because the
latent period is longer than the biological life of the pollutant residue.

SPECIFIC ENVIRONMENTAL FACTORS

RESPIRATORY DISEASES

Occupation

Acute respiratory diseases (Ammonia, chlorine inhala-
tions, zinc fumes) are emergencies and usually a clear history is available.

Chronic lung disease, however, may be clinically evident
long after the patient has left the occupation responsible
for his debilitation. This becomes important in diagnosis
but may also be relevant in terms of compensation. Coal
miners pneumococcosis is a serious widespread problem in
Appalachia. A study in 1969[16] showed that ten percent of
working miners and 20 percent of nonworking miners show

roentgenographic evidence of the disease. Exposure to low
level concentrations of a number of industrial dusts (alumi-
num, tin, cotton,[15] beryllium,[20] etc.) gives rise to diffuse
pulmonary fibrosis. In chronic lung disease, as in many
other disease processes, the etiological factors may be lost
unless they are carefully brought out in the history; and
even then, the proof may depend on clinical or epidemiological criteria and the exclusion of other causes. Silicosis,
for example, occurs in many trades - gold miners, metal
grinders, sandblasters; but pottery and ceramics also number
among the occupations where this dust may be a hazard. Of
particular importance is the frequent association between
tuberculosis and silicosis. The diagnosis of tuberculosis
should always include a thorough search for an environmental
contaminant which may facilitate the disease. Some infectious agents are associated with specific trades. Crypto-
strama corticale is a fungus found in dead wood, and stripping
of bark from maple logs liberates the spores giving rise to
acute respiratory illness - the Maple-bark Strippers Lung,
first described in 1932. Farmers Lung is another example of
an occupational hazard associated with a specific infectious
disease. This occurs among farmers in the midwest, who handle
mouldy grain or silage and who subsequently develop severe
dyspnea.[19]

NEUROLOGICAL DISEASES

The diagnosis of neurological disease presents a serious problem if a causative agent is not found. The presenting symptoms may be bizarre and the disease incorrectly labelled as viral or idiopathic. Yet it seems probable that many "idiopathic" diseases will ultimately be found to be due to common contaminants of our environment. Mercury is a case in point.

The tragic sequence of events of Minnemata, Japan, began with an onset of strange neurological signs - numbness, slurred speech, deafness, visual disturbances, ataxia, insomnia and emotional lability - that heralded the onset of a mystery disease (Kibyo) in this fishing community. Several years after the first signs manifested, it was established that the etiological agent was not a virus, but alkyl mercury from an industrial effluent released into the bay area. By that time, forty families had been affected and fifty lives lost.

Jamaica Ginger, a popular drink in the 1930's was found to be a cause of paralysis. This was a result of adding phosphorus, in the form of tri-ortho-cresyl-phosphate, to the drink. More recently phosphorus in the form of tetra-ethyl-pyrophosphate (TEPP) has proved to be a lethal contaminant of food. The organic phosphorus inhibits cholinesterase and death follows respiratory failure. Parathion,

another organo-phosphate commonly used as an insecticide,
has been shown to produce persistent EEG changes. <u>Insecti-
cides</u> may be insidious in their toxicity and give rise to
unexplained neuropathology. Recently cases of <u>impotence</u>
have been discovered to be associated with the use of organo-
phosphate insecticides. Previously held to be psychogenic
and frequently associated with long-standing diabetes
mellitus, impotence is another neurological symptom that
can be produced by an unsuspected environmental agent. Lead
has been mentioned as an example of an environmental poison
that appears in many forms. It is known to produce wrist
drop and cause encephalopathy in children. Sometimes an
alcoholic patient presenting with a wrist drop will be found
to be suffering from lead poisoning (lead contaminated moonshine) rather than alcoholic myopathy.

SKIN LESIONS

Environmental causes of skin lesions are common. They
include squamous carcinomas, associated with prolonged exposure to sunlight, found particularly in sensitive individuals
such as albinos. Occupational carcinomas occur on the lips
of sailors or fishermen who use their lips to mend their
nets. Other lesions may be bullae, ulcers or carcinomas from
man-made irradiation - x-rays or radioactive fallout. Iatrogenic causes of dermatitis vary from inorganic arsenicals,
previously used in the treatment of syphilis, to penicillin

reactions. Poison Ivy (Rhus toxicodendron) is one well
known irritant which produces dermatitis but there are innu-
merable other causes such as perfumes, plastics and insecticides.

CANCER

Occupational: Asbestos has been mentioned as a cause of
chronic lung disease.[17] It is also associated with lung
tumors, particularly mesotheliomas.[18] A diagnosis of meso-
thelioma should immediately suggest asbestos bodies. This
is not necessarily confined to mine workers, and the disease
may occur in persons only vaguely related to asbestos mining
such as local inhabitants of a mining town, construction
workers, pipe coverers or city dwellers not intimately con-
nected with any asbestos work but contaminated by asbestos
sprayed on girders as insulating material.

   Cancer of the bladder is another industrial hazard,
particularly in the aniline dye industry. It should not be
thought that this occupational hazard is under control. Cole
et al[6] recently emphasized the high incidence of bladder
cancer among leather workers and rubber workers. They also
point out that cooks and clerical workers are high risk populations for bladder cancer but in these groups since no
common carcinogen factor has been found, factors must be
sought in a common life style.

Any patient with cancer must have an occupational history taken since his disease may alert the physician to other
potential cases in the same occupation or in the same area.
Habitat: Domestic causes of cancers are not well defined.
However, homes with open fireplaces should be suspect particularly if the chimney is inadequate or nonexistent. Soot
on the walls is potentially carcinogenic. More widespread,
however, is the enormous load of polycylic aromatic hydrocarbons in the atmosphere of big cities. These carcinogens
are present in the unburnt emissions of domestic and industrial fires and in motor vehicle exhausts. There is considerable literature on the association between air pollution
and lung cancer.
Habits: Hydrocarbons are now associated with the toxic
effects found in "glue sniffers" who develop renal and liver
damage. They are also linked with the syndrome of "sudden
death" in young addicts. These compounds occur in many substances - spot removers solvents, plastic foams, glue, etc. -
which can readily be bought in drugstores, hardware stores
and garden shops. Since their effects may be relatively
innocuous in the early stage and the clinical presentation
unpredictable, a history of volatile fluids inhaled or swal-
lowed may be the only clue to the diagnosis.

The high incidence of cancer in cigarette smokers is
well documented. Cigarette smoke alone may not be carcinogen

but may be a co-factor or one of many in the pathogenesis of lung cancer. Thus city dwellers have a higher incidence of lung cancer than country folk, but smokers in cities have the highest incidence.

Tobacco in other forms is also carcinogenic. Tobacco chewers are prone to carcinoma of the buccal mucosa. Recently Baumslag et al showed that some snuff preparations in Swaziland (Africa) contain significant quantities of nickel and chromium, known carcinogenic agents. They suggested that these trace metals may be a factor in the high incidence of maxillary-antrum carcinomas among the African snuff sniffers and followed this up by reporting high concentrations of nickel and chrome in the soil in which the plants added to the snuff are grown.[2]

CARDIOVASCULAR DISEASES

At present, the major environmental factors known to be associated with myocardial infarction and atherosclerosis are cigarette smoking, air pollution (particularly CO) and trace metals.

The relationship between cigarette smoking and cardiovascular disease, like its association with lung cancer, is well documented. Less well appreciated is the fact that carbon monoxide, present in relatively high concentrations in busy city street, binds with hemoglobin to produce carboxymethhemoglobinemia - and this bond is not easily broken.

In addition, CO produces transient vasodilatation of the
coronary arteries.[10] Thus a city dweller, whose vasculature
is already the seat of atherosclerosis, rushing through a
carbon monoxide polluted area may suffer severe ischemia
not only as a result of his atheromatous vessels but because
the dilatation of those vessels and the reduced oxygen supply
compromise cardiac function. Cardiovascular problems should
always be discussed against the patient's environmental background if the treatment of the disease is to be complete
and further attacks successfully averted.

Trace metal studies link cadmium and zinc to cardiovascular disease and hypertension.[21] In assessing factors
that may be contributing to myocardial ischemia, dietary
intake other than cholesterol and saturated fats should come
up for consideration. Does the patient live in a soft water
area (soft water is thought to be associated with cardiovascular disease)? Does his diet contain a preponderance of
trace metals? Hemochromatosis may be induced by diet and
cardiac failure is a known cause of death in severe cases.
Is he a beer drinker and does the beer contain large amounts
of cobalt?[3]

Attention has been drawn to some environmental agents
which are known to be associated with disease. Every clinical
history needs to include careful attention to environmental
factors in food, drink and in the air we breathe. If the

physician is not aware of the ever present problem, he may

be lead to serious errors of judgment.

REFERENCES

1. Arean VM: Schistosomiasis: A clinicopathologic eval-
    uation. Pathology Annual, Vol. 1. Edited by SC
    Sommers. New York, Appleton-Century-Crofts, 1966

2. Baumslag N, Keen P: Trace elements in soil and plants
    and antral cancer. Arch Environ Health 25:23, 1972

3. Beer: With and without cobalt. Lancet 2:928, 1967

4. Bouhuys A, Barbero A, Schilling RSF, van de Woestigne
    KP: Chronic respiratory disease in hemp workers. Amer
    J Med 46:526, 1969

5. Blade E, Ferrand EF: Sulfur dioxide air pollution in
    New York City: Statistical analysis of twelve years.
    J Air Pollu Contr Ass 19:No. 11, 1969

6. Bregman JI: Man, water, and environment. Arch Environ
    Health 20:100, 1970

7. Coflin DL: Air pollution: Present and future threat
    to man and his environment. Advances in Environmental
    Science and Technology. Edited by Pitts, Metcals.
    New York, Wiley-Interscience, 1971

8. Cole P, Hoover R, Friedell GH: Occupation and cancer
    of the lower urinary tract. Cancer 29:1250, 1972

9. David O, Clark J, Kytja V: Lead and hypersensitivity.
    Lancet 2:900,1972

10. DeBias DA, Birkhead NC, Banerjee CM, Kazal LA, Holburn
    RR, Greene CH, Harrer WV, Rosenfeld LM, Menduke H,
    Williams N, Friedman MHF: Effects of chronic exposure
    to carbon monoxide on the cardiovascular and hematologic
    systems in dogs with experimental myocardial infarction.
    Int Arch Occup Health (Int Arch Arbeitsmed) 29:253, 1972

11. Ehrlich PR, Ehrlich AH: Population resources environ-
    ment. Second edition. San Francisco, W.H. Freeman and
    Company, 1972

12. Environmental hazards. Reprinted from New Eng J Med,
    Copyright, 1966, by the Massachusetts Medical Society.

13. Gaitan E, MacLenna R, Island DP, Liddle GW: Identifi-
    cation of water-borne goitrogens in the Cauca Valley

of Colombia. Trace Substances in Environmental Health,
Vol. V. Edited by DD Hemphill. Columbia, University
of Missouri, 1972

14. Hafen BQ: Man, Health and Environment. Minneapolis,
     Burgess Publishing Co., 1972

15. Hunter D: The Diseases of Occupation. Fourth edition.
     Boston, Little, Brown and Co., 1969

16. Lainhart WS, Doyle HN, Enterline PE, Henschel A, Ken-
     drick MA. Pneumoconiosis in Appalachian Bituminous
     Coal Miners. Public Health Service Publication No.
     2000. Cincinnati, USDHEW, PHS, Consumer Protection
     and Environmental Health Service, Environmental Control
     Administration, Bureau of Occupational Safety and
     Health, 1969

17. Selikoff IJ, Hammond EC: Community effects of non-
     occupational environmental asbestos exposure. Amer J
     Public Health 58:1658, 1968

18. Selikoff IJ, Bader RA, Bader ME, Churg J, Hammond EC:
     Asbestosis and neoplasia. Amer J Med 42:487, 1967

19. Spencer H: The pneumoconioses and other occupational
     lung diseases. Pathology of the Lung. Second edition.
     New York, Pergamon Press, 1968

20. Stoeckle JD, Hardy HL, Weber AL: Chronic berrylium
     disease. Amer J Med 46:545, 1969

21. Voors AW, Shuman MS, Gallagher PN: Atherosclerosis
     and hypertension in relation to some trace elements in
     tissues. To be published in World Rev Nutr and Diet,
     Vol. 15, 1973

22. Williams D, Williams WJ, Williams JE: Enzyme histo-
     chemistry of epithelioid cells in sarcoidosis and
     sarcoid-like gramulomas. J Path 97:705, 1959

23. Zapp JA: Man, air and environment. Arch Environ Health
     20:96, 1970

CHAPTER 12

Family Dentistry

ALAN DRINNAN

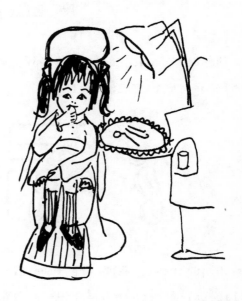

DENTAL CARIES (DECAY) and periodontal disease (gum disease) are two of the commonest diseases to affect the people in the United States and yet, paradoxically, these two diseases are poorly understood by most medical practitioners. Although the dental profession is responsible for the definitive treatment of disorders of the teeth and gums, the physician should know the signs and symptoms of the common oral diseases and be able to answer those questions which are frequently asked about the mouth and teeth. This chapter reviews basic facts about the teeth.

Some important topics are discussed and the chapter concludes
with questions concerning the teeth and mouth which are frequently asked of physicians.

THE TEETH

NUMBER, ERUPTION TIME, ETC.

The deciduous dentition (primary, first, baby or milk
teeth) consists of 20 teeth.

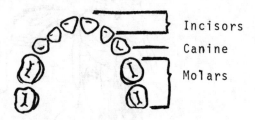

In each quadrant there are five teeth - one central incisor,
one lateral incisor, one canine tooth, a first molar and a
second molar. The following table shows the approximate
times of their eruption and exfoliation.

DECIDUOUS TEETH (20)

TOOTH	ERUPTION*	EXFOLIATION
Central Incisor	6 months	6-7 years
Lateral Incisor	9 months	6-7 years
Canine	18 months	9-11 years
First Molar	12 months	9-11 years
Second Molar	24 months	9-11 years

*It should be noted that there is a considerable variation
in the times of eruption of the deciduous teeth.

The exfoliation of deciduous teeth is a process which proceeds in "fits and starts". At times there is an active resorption of tooth substance followed by the deposition of new calcified material. This accounts for the fact that an exfoliating tooth may appear to be loose one day and yet more firm some days later. Occasionally, the process of exfoliation goes wrong. New calcified tissue is deposited on the root surface and joins with the jaw bone resulting in ankylosis of the tooth. Such a tooth does not exfoliate further. Prolonged retention of a milk tooth merits investigation by a dentist as it may be due to a variety of conditions, such as a missing successor or ankylosis.

The permanent dentition consists of 32 teeth.

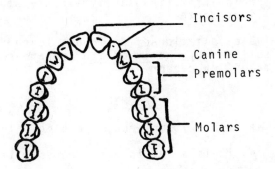

In each quadrant, the eight teeth are from midline - distally: central incisor, lateral incisor, canine (cuspid), first and second premolar (bicuspids), first, second and third molars.

The eruption times of these teeth are shown below.

PERMANENT TEETH (32)

TOOTH	ERUPTION
Central incisor	6-8 years
Lateral incisor	6-8 years
Canine	10-12 years
First premolar	10-12 years
Second premolar	10-12 years
First molar	6-7 years
Second molar	11-13 years
Third molar (wisdom tooth)	18-22 years

Note: 1. There is a very wide individual variation in the eruption times of teeth. The above table represents the average times although a delay of six months or even longer is not unusual.

2. Normally eruption proceeds the same bilaterally.

3. Mandibular teeth usually erupt just ahead of maxillary teeth.

4. The exfoliation of deciduous teeth is not always followed by the immediate appearance of the permanent successor.

TEETHING

Much has been written about teething pain. Many have said that, "As it is a physiologic process, it should not be painful." Such logic does not merit discussion as most mothers who have had children "per vias naturales" without the benefit of anesthesia will agree! Certainly the fact that children are erupting or shedding teeth from the age of about six months to thirteen years has been a convenient explanation of fever or malaise. Make sure that other causes

have been ruled out. Usually, apart from some slight irritation at the time the tooth is about to break through the oral
mucosa, there is little pain associated with teething. Sometimes the small flap of gum tissue (operculum) immediately
over a nearly erupted tooth may become inflamed and require
treatment. Occasionally, a small, bluish dome - an eruption
cyst - is seen over the crown of an erupting tooth. In most
cases, however, an eruption cyst will rupture and disappear
spontaneously. It is important that the physician has excluded an ear or throat infection and has looked at the mouth
properly before making the diagnosis of "teething" pain.

MIXED DENTITION

The period of mixed dentition, when teeth from the deciduous and permanent series are present together (normally
six through thirteen years), is an important time as many
parents harbor concerns about the apparent "crowding" of the
teeth and make mistakes about the eruption patterns. The
most common problems are:

1. Decay of the 6 year molar. The first permanent
    molar tooth (sometimes called the "six-year molar")
    erupts at about six years of age. It appears in
    the alveolar ridge posterior to the two deciduous
    molars and is not preceded by any other tooth. The
    tooth is considered by many parents to be a milk
    tooth and because it is believed that such a tooth

will "fall out anyway" parents often neglect to
seek attention when this tooth shows signs of decay. It is a most important tooth since it will
not be replaced. Because of its importance in
guiding development of the other molar teeth, and
particularly the relationship between neighboring
teeth and teeth in the other arch, it has been
called the "keystone"tooth of the dental arch.

2.   Overcrowding of the teeth. A second problem of
the mixed dentition is the appearance of "over
crowding". The teeth during the mixed dentition
are often very irregular in appearance and this
may cause concern to parents who have an under-
standable worry about a possible need for expensive
orthodontic treatment. Some cases of overcrowding
will sort themselves out without treatment and
others will require orthodontic intervention. A
dentist's opinion should be sought to discuss the
situation.

NUMBERING OF TEETH

There are several systems for numbering the teeth and
it is sufficient for the physician to know the most common
one in use in the United States at the present time. This
numbers the teeth sequentially starting on the patient's
right maxilla with the last molar tooth as #1, the second

right molar as #2, the first molar #3, and so on around to
the left side. The numbers then "drop" to the left mandible,
and the third molar there is #17, the second molar #18, and
so on around to the third molar on the right side which is
designated as #32. The system can be indicated:

```
1   2   3   4   5   6   7   8 |  9  10  11  12  13  14  15  16
32  31  30  29  28  27  26  25 | 24  23  22  21  20  19  18  17
```

The most usual system for designating the deciduous
dentition is using letters "a" through "e" in each quadrant
starting with the central incisor designated "a" and the
second deciduous molar as "e". The system is written:

```
e   d   c   b   a | a   b   c   d   e
e   d   c   b   a | a   b   c   d   e
```

CHARTING THE DENTAL RECORD

There are several methods of charting in use, some of
them involving anatomic diagrams of the teeth, others using
schematic figures.

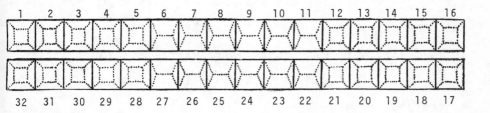

A dental record should indicate the teeth present, the location of any dental decay or fillings, the presence of gingivitis or periodontitis noting the depths of any pockets around
the teeth. A carious cavity is indicated by an open line

which delineates the extent of the cavity. Fillings are
shown by a "filled in" line. Examples of charting symbols
are shown below.

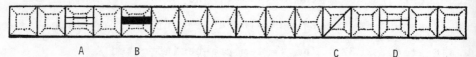

       A   B   C   D

A: Cavity present
B: Filling
C: Tooth for extraction
D: Tooth missing

ANOMALIES IN THE NUMBER OF TEETH

    Occasionally, a child will fail to develop the full num-
ber of teeth (anodontia or oligodontia). This is more likely
to happen in the permanent than in the deciduous dentition.
Some cases of missing teeth may be associated with other
developmental anomalies, e.g. the condition of ectodermal
dysplasia in which the hair, sweat glands and fingernails
may be involved. In a few instances, a familial pattern can
be determined, but often missing a tooth or teeth affects a
single individual and his siblings or children do not show
the same variation. The most usually missing tooth is a
third molar, the next a maxillary lateral incisor (particularly in females) and then the maxillary or mandibular
second premolars.

SUPERNUMERARY TEETH

    Occasionally, a person develops teeth in addition to
the usual complement of 32 permanent teeth. The most common
site for an extra tooth is in the anterior region of the

maxilla. Fourth molars and extra premolars are sometimes
seen. There are a few cases of people with a third dentition on record, but these were probably people with many
supernumerary teeth.

VARIATIONS IN THE DEVELOPMENT OF THE TEETH

The variations which are probably the best known to the
physician are those occurring in congenital syphilitics -
Hutchinsons's incisors and mulberry molars. The Hutchinson's
incisor teeth occur in the permanent dentition. A typical
tooth shows a narrowing of the width of the incisal edge
with, frequently, a central notching of the incisal margin.
The shape of the tooth has been likened to a screwdriver
blade and the term "screwdriver incisor" has been used.

NORMAL INCISOR   HUTCHINSON'S INCISOR

The first permanent molar tooth of the congenital syphilitic may show a very irregular surface. The normal cusp
pattern is lost and many irregular mounds of enamel cover
the surface. The resemblance of this "bumpy" surface to a
mulberry accounts for the name.

In certain other conditions the teeth do not develop
correctly and hypoplastic teeth may result. Diseases which
affect the teeth include those in which the calcium and

phosphorus levels in the blood are altered, endocrine disturbances, nutritional problems (such as Vitamin D deficienc
and possibly prolonged fevers. Once developmental defects
are incorporated into the teeth, there is little that can
be done to rectify them. It is important that children with
such problems receive regular dental care so that all necessary dental restorative measures can be performed early.

TETRACYCLINE STAINING OF TEETH

Drugs of the tetracycline series can be incorporated
into developing teeth and bones, and, if administered over
a long period of time during which a child's teeth are developing, may cause unpleasant staining of the teeth. This
staining cannot be removed and a child may be quite concerned about the "dirty" teeth. The condition is likely to
be seen in children who have suffered from chronic infection
and who have been given tetracyclines over a long period,
for example, children with cystic fibrosis. In any serious
illness where tetracycline is the drug of choice, the fact
that some discoloration of the teeth may result is not likel
to contraindicate the use of the drug. However, where prolonged use of an antibiotic is expected and an alternative
drug to tetracycline is available, it is suggested that this
alternative be used. Fully formed and calcified teeth are
not affected by tetracycline drugs.

DENTAL CARIES

Although the precise nature of dental caries is not
understood fully, the following summarizes the most important features of the disease.

Bacterial action on the carbohydrates which cling to
the tooth surfaces results in acid and enzyme formation.
The acid demineralizes the tooth substance and initiates the
breakdown of the tooth with eventual cavity formation. Generally there is a direct relationship between caries incidence and carbohydrate intake, poor oral hygiene and the
eating of sticky foods between meals.

The most common sites for food stagnation are the pits
and fissures on the occlusal (biting) and buccal (cheek)
surfaces, the areas of the tooth near the gum margin and
those places between the teeth (the interdental areas). Each
of these places may be easily overlooked if the teeth are
not brushed carefully. The stagnation can be readily visualized by staining the debris with a red dye released from
a tablet which the patient chews. The use of these "dis-
closing" tablets is becoming very common with the realiza-
tion by more and more dentists that much dental disease can
be prevented simply by having their patients practice very
careful oral hygiene.

Because early carious lesions are painless it is not
unusual for a patient to wait until the development of pain

before seeking dental advice. Dental pain may be of many
types, dull, sharp, transient, lingering, intensified by
cold, relieved by heat and so on. The type of pain is often
an indication of the extent of the decay. Patients complaining of dental pain should be seen by a dentist. The
physician should realize that many patients mistakenly consider their teeth to be the cause of facial pain, whereas
the pain may be arising from diseases of such related structures as the maxillary sinus, temporamandibular joint,
parotid gland, etc.

RAMPANT DENTAL CARIES

Rampant dental caries is frequently seen in young children. Many teeth "rot" away and soft black roots are all
that remain. This condition is common in low-income group
children and may result from poor oral hygiene measures or
dietary habits. Continued use of a feeding bottle containing
milk or fluids such as sweetened orange juice may lead to
rampant caries sometimes called "feeding bottle" or "milk
bottle" caries.

FLUORIDE AND TEETH

Fluoride is an essential trace element. It has several
known essential metabolic functions but, by far, the effect
on the dentition is best known.

Several well controlled studies have shown that children who grow up in a community in which the water supply

has a certain content of fluoride are less susceptible to
dental decay than children raised in an area in which the
water contains little or no fluoride. The precise mode of
action of fluoride is not known and several theories have
been suggested. It is known, for instance, that fluoride
may be incorporated into the hydroxyapatite crystal structure of the dental tissues and this fluoro-hydroxyapatite
crystal may be more resistant to the carious process. The
optimum level of fluoride in water is of the order of one
part per million and ingestion of water of this fluoride
concentration throughout all or most of the time that a
child is developing teeth provides maximum resistance to
dental caries. Many communities have naturally fluoridated
water supplies and others artificially fluoridate theirs.
Fluoride can be incorporated into developing teeth not only
by the ingestion of fluoridated water but by taking fluoride
tablets. The more reliable method of the two is the con-
tinuous ingestion of fluoridated water. Where natural fluoridation is deficient then artificial fluoridation of municipal water supplies should be made. Fluoride can be absorbed
onto the surface layers of erupted teeth following the direct
application of fluoridated toothpaste or sodium fluoride
solutions but the protection offered by this method is less
satisfactory. In areas where fluoride content of the water
is high, dental mottling may occur.

PERIODONTAL DISEASE

Periodontal disease (a disease of the supporting tissues of the teeth) is very common and is the most important cause of lost teeth in adults. More teeth are lost as the result of periodontal disease than for any other reason. The disease is believed to start as a result of the formation of various enzymes and toxins in the gingival crevice. These substances produce inflammatory changes in the periodontium. Destruction of the collagen fibers which support the teeth leads to the development of pocketing around the teeth. These pockets can harbor food, bacterial and cellular debris and these then act as the source of further destructive substances. Unfortunately, most cases of periodontal disease are chronic and patients are unaware that there is anything wrong. In many cases, a superficial oral examination may suggest that the teeth and gums are healthy. The gums do not look inflamed and the patient does not complain of any particular problem. It is only when the depths of the gum crevices are probed, the mobility of the teeth evaluated and the bone supporting the teeth visualized by x-rays that the disease can be detected and evaluated accurately.

It is important to remember that many patients with advanced periodontal disease have no symptoms and it is only when the disease produces loosening and drifting of their teeth that patients realize something is wrong. Because of the high incidence of the disease and the early "symptomless" stage, it is recommended that all adults have periodic dental examinations.

PREGNANCY AND DENTISTRY

The old adage, "For every child, you lose a tooth", is not true. Fully developed teeth are not a source of minerals in dietary deficiency, osteomalacia or pregnancy. Any increased susceptibility to dental caries during pregnancy is more likely to be the result of external factors such as less attention to oral hygiene rather than a change in tooth calcification. Bone minerals can be mobilized when required and alveolar bone may be demineralized in a deficiency state.

Gingival changes occurring in pregnancy are quite common and the condition of "pregnancy gingivitis" is well recognized. The gingivae are particularly vascular and hyperplastic. They bleed easily and in some cases, quite discrete hyperplastic growths are seen arising from the gingival margin or the interdental gingival area. These have been called "pregnancy" tumors. The histological changes in these "tumors" are not those of a malignant condition but rather show inflammatory, vascular hyperplasia. Most cases of "pregnancy tumor" or "pregnancy gingivitis" are seen in patients with poor oral hygiene. The best treatment is prophylactic and all pregnant patients should be sure to have dental advice and care throughout pregnancy.

Few problems develop with the teeth of the fetus if the mother is receiving a well balanced diet. The teeth start to develop at about six weeks after conception and mineralization begins soon after. Frequently mothers will ask about the need to take extra calcium or vitamin tablets during their pregnancies "to ensure baby has good teeth". Providing a mother is taking an adequate diet for general development, there is no particular indication to give her more vitamins or minerals just for the child's teeth.

Most dental services can be provided during pregnancy, but it is important to encourage women to see their dentists regularly to avoid the need for any involved dental treatment during a pregnancy.

TRAUMATIC INJURY TO THE TEETH

It is not unusual for children to damage their teeth or the soft tissues of the mouth. Children who often place objects in their mouths may stumble, and cause lacerations of the soft tissues or they may fall and fracture some teeth. The extent of such injuries is very variable and the prognosis for a case will depend often on the child receiving prope attention as soon as possible. Injuries to the mouth often produce much bleeding and swelling and may be a source of great anxiety to the child and his parents. Dental injuries may vary from a slight chip of the enamel edge of a tooth to the complete displacement of a tooth from its socket.

Fortunately, most of such injuries can be managed perfectly well by a competent dentist, who, by using certain restorative techniques, and splinting procedures, can usually achieve a satisfactory cosmetic and functional result. If a physician is called to examine a child who has a fractured tooth or a lacerated lip, he should examine the child very carefully to be certain that he does not overlook any other injury. If a tooth is fractured or missing, then the possibility of the tooth or a fragment of the tooth being lodged in the oral soft tissues must be remembered. On occasion, a lip or buccal mucosal laceration has been cleaned and sutured over a hidden tooth fragment. In some circumstances a totally displaced tooth may be re-implanted and many cases reporting the successful retention of such teeth have appeared in the literature. It is not sufficient to simply clean the tooth and insert it back into the socket! The tooth requires special treatment before being replaced. The pulp chamber of the tooth must be cleaned and then filled so that any "dead space" that could harbor necrotic debris and bacteria is obliterated. Any replantation should be done by a dentist. If a physician is given a dislodged tooth or can locate one at the site of an accident, he should keep it in a clean sponge and give it to the dentist as soon as possible. On rare occasions teeth that have been dislodged have been aspirated and this possibility should always be considered

in those people who develop respiratory signs or symptoms
after a facial injury involving the loss of teeth.

ORAL ULCERS

Recurrent oral ulceration (canker sores or aphthous
ulcers) is a very common affliction of unknown etiology.
The lesions are sometimes referred to as herpes ulcers, but
in the vast majority of cases, no positive evidence of herpes
virus infection can be found. Fortunately, the majority of
ulcers heal with or without treatment within seven to ten
days. It has been said, facetiously, that the actively
treated ulcers take one to one and one half weeks to heal,
whereas the untreated ulcers will heal in seven to ten days!

The lesions may be single or multiple and present as
painful, sharply defined ulcers with a necrotic slough on
the surface and an erythematous zone around them. There is
no definitive treatment available. The preparation orabase
emollient which is an adhesive substance which sticks to the
mucosal surface, is useful for covering these sensitive ul-
cerated areas.

SORE MOUTH - STOMATITIS

There are many reasons why a patient may complain of a
sore mouth. One form of herpes virus infection - primary
herpetic gingivostomatitis - may affect children or adults
and result in ulceration of the gingivae, oral and pharyngeal
ulceration, fever and cervical lymphadenopathy. There is no

definitive "anti-herpes" treatment for this condition and the management is symptomatic - relief of pain and prevention of secondary infection.

Trench mouth, also known as necrotizing ulcerative gingivitis or Vincent's infection, occurs most usually in young adults especially in those with "neglected" mouths. The condition presents as a painful gingivitis characterized by necrosis of the gingival margins, a marked foetor oris and elevation of temperature. The treatment nearly always requires careful attention to the gingivae and in some cases antibiotic therapy. It is most important that patients with the condition seek dental advice to prevent recurrent bouts of the disease.

A common finding in old people, particularly women, is glossodynia - a condition in which the patient has a red, atrophic, smooth tongue and suffers the sensation of burning in the tongue (glossopyrosis). This condition is frequently associated with nutritional disorders, hormonal changes, iron deficiency (with or without anemia) and sometimes Candida infection (Moniliasis). Each of these possibilities and "local" factors such as ill fitting dentures, or sensitivity to denture materials must be considered when evaluating a complaint of a "sore mouth" in an older patient. Physicians should seek advice from their dental colleagues if in any doubt.

VITAMIN C AND GINGIVITIS

Vitamin C deficiency may be associated with the development of swollen, easily bleeding gingivae. The condition is
not common in the United States today, although it is occasionally seen in patients who may have neglected their diets
for such reasons as alcoholism or food fadism.

DILANTIN

Fibrous enlargement of the gingivae is an occasional
side effect seen in patients receiving Dilantin (diphenylhydantoin sodium). The gingivae may become extremely hyperplastic and almost cover the teeth. The degree of hyperplasia
can be kept to a minimum if the patient receives regular
dental attention.

DENTURE WEARING

There are many millions of Americans who have lost their
natural teeth and have had their dentitions restored by the
provision of prosthetic appliances. The development of reliable, non-irritative materials has meant that the majority
of patients can wear dentures satisfactorily and suffer little
inconvenience from having lost their natural teeth. There
are few cases of nutritional deficiency which can be blamed
on a defective dentition. There is such a wide range of
soft foods available and so many people have blenders that
few people go short of essential foodstuffs because of any
difficulty in wearing dentures. It is not advocated that

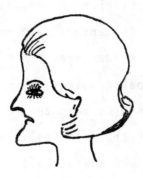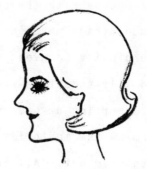

Without Teeth   With Teeth

dentures are unnecessary. They have important functions in
addition to mastication - speech, appearance, and so on. It
is certainly better that solid foods be masticated.

It must be remembered that the jaws are changing constantly. Following the extraction of teeth, the supporting
or alveolar bone resorbs to leave a smooth, edentulous ridge.
Most of this shrinkage occurs in the first few months following extractions but there continues to be a gradual altering of the contour of the ridges throughout life - the
degree of shrinkage varies. Many people who have dentures
immediately following extractions are told that their dentures are a "temporary" set and they will have a permanent
set later on. This gives the patient an erroneous idea.
Dentures should never be considered permanent. It is essential that patients with dentures return to their dentist
every few years for evaluation. It is quite possible for a
denture to become loose and cause considerable irritation of

the oral mucosa with the proliferation of hyperplastic tissue. Such tissue makes an unstable denture base and may need
to be surgically removed before new dentures can be con-
structed. If a denture-wearing patient seeks a physician's
advice concerning a sore in the mouth, then the physician
must examine the mouth first with the dentures in place and
then with them out. All too often mistakes have been made
by:

1.   Assuming that an ulcer was neoplastic, whereas,
      in fact, it was an inflammatory ulcer produced by
      an ill-fitting denture.

2.   Considering that an ulcer was a traumatic one
      when, in fact, it was a cancer.

The location of any oral ulcer and its relationship to
a denture edge, broken tooth or denture clasp must always
be evaluated. In the event that any of these potential irritants may have caused inflammation of the tissues, it is
necessary to remove the irritant and to confirm that there
is evidence of healing of the ulcer within one to two weeks.
Any inflammatory ulcer should begin to show evidence of
healing when the irritant which produced it is removed. A
neoplastic ulcer will continue to develop even if a suspected irritation is removed.

ORAL CANCER

The oral cavity may be the site of many types of cancer arising from any of the tissues normally present in the mouth (including the dental apparatus) or from remote tissues which have metastasized to the jaws or soft tissues.

Remember that any <u>swelling of the jaw</u>, <u>development of paresthesia of the face</u> or <u>loosening of teeth</u> might be evidence of a tumor and, in such cases, the patient should be referred to a dentist for evaluation.

The most serious oral neoplasm is squamous cell carcinoma. It represents about three to four per cent of all cancers. In 1970, it was estimated that 6,950 deaths occurred attributable to cancer of the oral cavity and pharynx. Most cases of intraoral cancer occur on the tongue. The posterior lateral border of the tongue and under surface should always be inspected and palpated during any oral examination.

Oral cancer may present as an ulcer, a red or white patch or as an exophytic growth. In their early stages, many cancers are painless and patients are unaware of them. Later they may metastasize to regional lymph nodes and in these cases the prognosis is much poorer than when the lesions remain localized. Oral cancer occurs more commonly in men than in women and although cases have been reported at all ages - even in children, the most usual age groups are 50 to 60 or older. Predisposing factors are thought to be

chronic oral infection, syphilitic glossitis, excessive use
of tobacco or snuff, and there appears to be an association
between oral cancer and cirrhosis of the liver. Any oral
ulceration which appears suspicious of malignancy should be
evaluated by a dentist or some specialist such as a head and
neck surgeon.

QUESTIONS COMMONLY ASKED BY PARENTS
At What Age Should I Take My Child to the Dentist?

A child should be taken to a dentist as early as possible after the teeth have begun to erupt and certainly not
later than two to two and one half years. This familiarizes
the child with the dentist's office, personnel, instruments
and procedures. If a child's first dental visit is made
because of pain, his later acceptance of dental care is not
likely to be so pleasant.
How Often Should a Child Visit the Dentist?

To prevent dental disease the child should be taken to
the dentist at least once every six months and, of course,
at other times if there is evidence of bleeding gums, pain,
swelling, or any other sign or symptom of dental disease.
At What Age Should a Child Practice Oral Hygiene?

As early as is possible. Children vary in their ability
to handle a toothbrush but should be encouraged to clean
their teeth as soon as they are able. The mother, of course,
should clean their gums and the teeth as soon as they erupt.

Restrict refined carbohydrate to mealtimes. Children should
be taught to rinse the mouth regularly after eating.

If possible, the teeth should be brushed within 15
minutes after each meal in a definite order:

1.   Chewing surfaces upper and lower teeth
2.   Outside surface upper teeth
3.   Inside surface upper teeth
4.   Outside surface lower teeth
5.   Inside surface lower teeth

The bristles should point to the roots first and they should
sweep over the gums towards the biting surface of the teeth.

Will Thumbsucking Cause a Permanent Deformity to a Child's Jaw?

Persistent thumbsucking into the teens may cause distortion in the normal development of the jaws. Fortunately,
although nearly all children go through a stage of thumbsucking very few continue the habit long enough to cause any
permanent distortion to their teeth and jaws.

At What Age Should Active Measures Be Taken to Discourage Thumbsucking?

There is no precise answer to this question as so much
depends on the individual child, general physiological and
psychological development, emotional maturity and so on. A
dental consultation should be arranged if there is any doubt
in the physician's mind about the possibility of any jaw
deformity developing.

Can Some Families Have "Poor" Teeth?

There are inherited diseases which predispose to "gum trouble" or "poor or soft teeth" but they are uncommon. When several members of a family appear predisposed to dental decay and/or periodontal problems such as gingivitis (inflammation of the gums) or periodontitis (inflammation of the supporting structures of the teeth - periodontal ligament and bone) it is likely that this predisposition results from environmental factors. A poor family diet (for example - too many sticky foods), the habit of eating snacks between meals, poor oral hygiene practices (infrequent or no toothbrushing) are factors which probably affect each member of a family. In most cases, when attempting to evaluate poor oral health in a family, these causes should be considered more likely than inherited defects in the structure of the teeth and periodontal tissues.

REFERENCES

1.   Burket: Oral Medicine. Sixth edition. Philadelphia,
     J.B. Lippincott and Company, 1971

2.   Glickman J: Review of periodontal disease. New Eng
     J of Med 284:1071, 1972

3.   Keyes P: Review of research in dental caries. J of
     Amer Dental Assoc 76:1357, 1968

4.   Zegarelli, Kutscher, Hyman: Diagnosis of Diseases of
     the Mouth and Jaws. Philadelphia, Lea and Febiger,
     1969

CHAPTER 13

Family Records

IRVING KANNER

EXCELLENT MEDICAL CARE requires excellent medical records. These must be adequate and legible to all who may need to use them in the patient's care or for later review. Nothing should be trusted to the physician's memory.

The record traditionally has been structured to source orientation, i.e., different parts of the record were grouped together depending on the source. Laboratory work was kept in one place, hospital summaries in another. In the hospital chart separate sections had been kept for nurses notes, physiotherapy, physicians orders, progress notes, etc. Buried at the end of the work-up the physician had placed his impressions. The orders may have followed here, or on a special sheet, in no special order, often helter-skelter. The nurse could not always determine which order was for which problem. A very lengthy record was often nearly useless.

Lawrence Weed[6] pioneered a new structure for organization and use of medical records. The concept is known as
the Problem Oriented Medical Record (POMR). His aim was to
bring order to the record, make it a useful tool for following the patient's course and allow intelligent review and
criticism. He planned a record that would be an instrument
for teaching and would thus improve patient care. In the
POMR the individual problems of the patient are detailed,
including pertinent history and findings, both physical and
laboratory (including x-ray). The assessment and the plans
for each problem (diagnostic, therapeutic, and educational)
are enumerated individually. This is particularly of value
for a patient with many problems. Bjorn and Cross[1], who
worked with him, use Weed's ideas in their semi-rural family
practice in Maine. With flow sheets and problem lists, they
have succeeded in having records that reflect the patient's
progress and can easily be reviewed and audited. Hurst and
Walker of Emory have championed the cause of POMR and successfully introduced it into Atlanta. Their recent book[3]
is an excellent in depth review of the method.

Combining the problem oriented record with modern
methods of medical data collection should help produce
efficient and dynamic delivery of health care. Earlier in
this volume, there have been a number of suggestions for
data gathering and charting.

The Problem Oriented Medical Record utilizes the patient's data base for development of the problem list and
plan. Follow-up records can often be kept in graphic form
to save time.

I.   The Data Base - best defined by age, sex, sub-specialty
      and often by presenting problem. It consists of the
      patient's medical history, physical examination and
      routine laboratory and x-ray studies.

      A.   Taking the medical history

           1.   Present Illness: Obtaining the history of
                the present illness requires a simple, direct
                approach. No computer program is as effective
                as an interested listener. Though often pre-
                ceeded by a business like, but warm greeting,
                the opening gambit is the interviewer's ques-
                tion, "What is the problem that brought you
                here today?" This may only produce a useless
                response, such as "my wife brought me", or
                "It's been several years since I've had a
                checkup and just thought it was time for it".
                The interviewer must not accept these answers,
                but must persist until he finds the actual
                reason the patient has come. The visit may
                have been provoked by such an event as a
                neighbor's sudden heart attack causing

patient's concern over a previously slight
chest distress.

After the patient's chief complaint has been
ascertained, questions are asked primarily to
start the patient talking - reinforcing, when
necessary, with an understanding gesture or
word to keep the patient talking. If the patient hesitates, repeating the last word or
phrase with a rising inflection may be a useful ploy. Further questions are asked to
determine when the various symptoms started
and their progression to the present. The
severity and detailed character of the symptoms, the effect of therapy, both home remedies
and that given by professionals is sought.
The relationship of the symptoms to other
events, both social and physical, is ascertained. Contacts are important in communicable diseases. Relationship to meals or
foods, or symptoms that awaken the patient
from sleep should be noted.

Some patients will pour out their problems in
profusion and with much detail. Do not judge
too quickly that this is all on an emotional
basis. Let the patient ventilate as much as

possible, taking only enough notes so you can go back over each of the problems later. Yarnell calls this the "Problem History".[7]

2.   Past History, Systems Review, Family History, Social History (This is Yarnell's Data Base History[7])

These portions of the history are best obtained with the help of some form of questionnaire, preferably answered by the patient. The aid of a family member or a trained assistant may be required. Although experiments are being performed with patients interacting with computers through a terminal, such methods are still too expensive for routine office use. Pencil and paper questionnaires are more economical and practical in most situations. Examples are the Cornell Medical Index[2] and the Programmed Medical History (PMH)[4] and Medical History Screen (PMH-S). The first requires no processing, the second and third can be processed with ordinary office equipment or with a computer. Other questionnaires are available commercially. The print-out of the programmed history can be read and verified quickly, saving

much physician time. If you are to take
these portions of the history yourself, you
must learn to do so in a systematic way, or
you will omit essential portions. It is wise
to have a preplanned format of questions. If
the questions are written in outline in tele-
graphic style, the outline can be typed or
printed on one side of a single page. This
can be laid on the desk for a guide. An outline for general adult medicine is shown
(Figure 13.1, page 310).

B.   Recording the physical examination. This can be
done long hand, or if available, the Programmed
Physical Examination (PPE)[5] may be used. The main
questions of the PPE are a useful guide (Figure
13.2, page 312).

C.   Sum up the lab and x-ray data already reported.

D.   A complete work-up is not required on the first
visit (which may be for a specific complaint) but
should be planned for all who are to continue
being your patients.

II. Problem List

A.   From this data base, the examiner must extract
every problem and make up a numbered problem list
which is current and complete. The problems should

be listed only at the height of definition that is possible at the moment, based upon the data obtained. By this we mean, no "guess" diagnoses are to be included, no "rule-out" diagnoses, but instead, if all we know at the moment is that the patient is complaining of a headache and nothing more, then the problem is "headache". If we have found elevated blood pressure but have not found whether this is a sustained reading, or the cause of it, we don't write "essential hypertension" but instead write "elevated blood pressure". If a laboratory result is abnormal and the cause of it has not been determined, such as an elevated blood sugar, we may only write for the problem "hyperglycemia". Should we have a physiological finding, such as congestive failure, for which we have not yet found the cause, then it is simply written on the problem list "congestive failure, etiology undetermined". Include all problems, such as social, demographic, or emotional. Inactive problems are to be so indicated.

B.   It is probably wisest, on the first visit, to list these problems, following the gathering of the data base, using pencilled letters (A,B,C) rather than numerically and then the following day (or on

the next visit, in the case of an outpatient) to
review and make up the permanent problem list, re-
placing the letters with numbers. By this time
the doctor has had a chance to get some additional
laboratory work and some time to think and read.
The problem that brought the patient to medical
attention is marked with an asterisk. All active
problems are followed with an arrow. The permanent
problem list should be placed in the front of the
chart and should look like that shown in Figure
13.3. It should be on fairly heavy-stock paper.
As greater sophistication in the knowledge of the
problem is acquired, a more definitive statement
of the problem is added, until, finally, it is in
the form of a diagnosis when this is possible. It
will be noted that the problem list has a place
for the date each problem was first entered. When
the problem becomes inactive or is resolved, the
date of this explanatory progress note is written
above the arrow. Since the chart follow-up notes
are dated, these references to the date of diagnosis and resolution of problem make the numbered
problem list act as a table of contents of the chart

C.   If the data base is incomplete we now add a Problem
      "0" at the top of problem list - "IDB" (Incomplete

Figure 13.3

UNIVERSITY HOSPITAL
ALBERT B. CHANDLER MEDICAL CENTER
LEXINGTON, KENTUCKY

COMPLETE PROBLEM LIST
(Permanent Part of Medical Record)

*PHYSICIAN – Place * beside reason for admission*   *Imprint Area*

DATE ENTERED	PROBLEM NUMBER	ACTIVE	INACTIVE
10/15/70	1	Headaches ⟶ 3/1/71	Iatrogenic (Anovulatory drug)
2/1/71	2	Hypertension ⟶ 3/1/71	Iatrogenic (Anovulatory drug)
2/1/71	3	Hyperglycemia ⟶ 3/1/71 Chemical Diabetes Mellitus ⟶	

Data Base). As this problem is resolved, by completion, it is updated (Figure 13.4).

D.   In due time new problems may be the main reason
for treatment and will be marked with an asterisk.
Older asterisks are marked with a circle (Figure
13.4).

E.   Dr. William Daines of Ogden, Utah, suggests writing
below the arrow the part of the chart showing the
evidence, such as FS for Flow Sheet, PN for Progress Note, L for Lab, etc.

F.   If a previously inactivated problem recurs, an
arrow is drawn to the left to indicate this and
again appropriately dated. Skipping lines between
each problem listed will leave room for this even-
tuality.

G.   Should the problem recur very frequently it would
be well to consider resolving the title to "repeated _____" and to keep it active with dates
of the chart entries indicated.

H.   There are various ways suggested to enter minor
illnesses. Some keep these on a separate problem
list unless they are unusually frequent, when they
are entered as in G above. I prefer to enter URI
or GI upset, etc. on the regular problem list, and
treat as in G above if warranted.

Figure 13.4

UNIVERSITY HOSPITAL
ALBERT B. CHANDLER MEDICAL CENTER
LEXINGTON, KENTUCKY

COMPLETE PROBLEM LIST
(Permanent Part of Medical Record)

*PHYSICIAN – Place * beside reason for admission*   *Imprint Area*

DATE ENTERED	PROBLEM NUMBER	ACTIVE	INACTIVE
8/1/72	0	IDB ————————— 8/4/72 Completed —————	→
		Pelvic 8/3/72 ↗	
		Rectal 8/3/72 ↗	
		EKG 8/4/72 ↗	
		Note the use of arrows--all active problems are followed with an arrow. When that problem is resolved (this can be to higher state of definition, to inactivity, or found to be a part of another problem) the date of resolution is written above the arrow and defined as indicated. Examples:	
7/5/71	1	ⓐ Edema —7/6/71→ CHF —7/8/71→ Coronary Thrombosis →	
8/3/72	2	* Abdominal distress —8/4/72→ Acute Appendicitis —8/4/72→	S/P Appendectomy

III. <u>Plan List</u>. On the initial problem list, which was tem-
porarily numbered with letters for each problem, a plan
with the same letter of the alphabet will be marked
down. Plan A is for Problem A, Plan B for Problem B,
etc. (If numbers are used from the start, then Plan 1
is for Problem 1, Plan 2 for Problem 2, etc.). The
plan list for each problem should include any further
requirements in the way of procedures for diagnoses and
here we can include such statements as "rule out 'X'
disease". Unlike our old-fashioned charts, we are required here to say how we are going to rule out 'X'
disease and what parameters will allow us to rule it
out. For example we mentioned hyperglycemia. We may
say we are going to rule out diabetes mellitus by feeding
the patient an adequate sugar diet for so many days,
followed by a glucose tolerance test and that if the
blood sugar is less than 160 mgm/100 cc. after eating
and is back to normal (pre-glucose load) at two hours,
then we shall have ruled out diabetes. The next part
of the plan list for each problem would be any therapeutic measures to be taken and what parameters will be
judged to indicate therapeutic effect or toxicity. For
example, if this patient were to be a diabetic, we might
specify the diet the patient is to have with a goal of
80% of his blood sugars two hours p.c. being below 130

and if they are not, we will entertain the use of hypoglycemic agents, such as insulin. The third part of
the plan for each problem would include those measures
taken for patient or family instruction, such as,
"Patient to be instructed in her diet, in the giving
of insulin, urine testing for sugar and acetone, and
hygienic care of the feet". Here is noted whether the
patient or family has been told the diagnosis and, if
pertinent, the prognosis (Figure 13.5).

IV.   Progress Notes. Progress notes shall be numbered and
titled according to the problem list. Each problem
that is going to be gone into at that visit will be mentioned separately. The format of that progress note
can be described as SOAP:

S is symptomatic. How the patient feels concerning
that problem, the history.

O is objective for the objective findings on the
examination concerning that problem. Include the
results of any laboratory procedures ordered under
the plans of the previous visit.

A is assessment. This could include the impression,
what we have ruled out, or the prognosis.

P is plans. Here again the plans are divided into
those necessary for further diagnostic studies, therapeutic and educational for the patient or the family
(Figure 13.6, page 303).

Figure 13.5

Young woman seen with complaint of <u>headaches</u> of four months duration, present on awakening in morning and lasting till after breakfast. Has been on birth control pills for six months. Physical examination showed only a <u>blood pres-</u><u>sure</u> elevation to 194/120, lab was negative except for <u>blood</u> <u>sugar</u> of 164, 2 hrs. p.c.

2/1/71   Problem:

1.   Headaches, etiology unknown

2.   Hypertension, etiology unknown

3.   Hyperglycemia

Plan:

1.   Headaches - Dx. Rule out birth control pills
      as cause by stopping. If headaches persist,
      get skull x-ray, EEG, consider brain scan.

      Rx. Diaphragm fitted (size 70 coil spring).

2.   Hypertension - Dx. Rule out birth control pill
      as in #1 by stopping them. If hypertension
      persists, get colony count urinalysis, hyper-
      tensive I.V.P., Serum K, V.M.A.

3.   Hyperglycemia - Dx. Rule out birth control
      pills as precipitant of chemical diabetes.
      When off pills get Glucose Tolerance Test.

Figure 13.6

Sample Progress Notes:

2/15/71   1.   Headaches:
                Subjective: Considerably improved in past 3
                               days.
                Objective: No findings. BP 160/100.
                Assessment: Probably iatrogenic - birth con-
                               trol pills.
                Plan: Continue off pill.

           2.   Hypertension:
                Subjective: None
                Objective: BP 160/100.
                Assessment: Iatrogenic - birth control pills.
                Plan: Continue off pills.

           3.   Hyperglycemia:
                Subjective: None
                Objective: Blood sugar 2 hrs. p.c. 110.
                Assessment: Possible subclinical chemical
                               diabetes, precipitated by use of
                               birth control pills.
                Plan: GTT next visit.

3/1/71   1.   Headaches:
                Subjective: Completely subsided 2 weeks.
                Objective: No finding.
                Assessment: Iatrogenic - "the pill".
                Plan: Avoid anovulatory Rx - Patient
                               instructed as to reason and
                               fitted with size 70 coil spring
                               diaphragm.

           2.   Hypertension:
                Subjective: None
                Objective: BP 120/78
                Assessment: Iatrogenic - "the pill".
                Plan: Avoid anovulatory Rx.

           3.   Hyperglycemia:
                Subjective: None.
                Objective: GTT shows sugar intolerance with
                               2 hr. glucose of 164, 3 hours 110
                                and 2+ in urine at 2 and 3 hours.
                Assessment: Chemical diabetes.
                Plan: Education of patient re: diet
                               (mod CHO restriction). Recheck
                               blood sugar 2 hrs. p.c. every 3 mos.

Not every problem will be discussed on each visit. Certainly problem #1 (which should have been the problem that brought the patient into the physician or hospital) should not be lost in the shuffle because problem #3 seems more important to the examiner at the moment. For example, "a patient came in complaining of headaches, and the physician found an elevated blood sugar. After many visits, the physician finally reassures the patient that he doesn't have diabetes and the patient says, "Well, Dr., I didn't think I had that, but what about my headache?" This should not occur with properly kept and used problem oriented medical records.

V. Flow Sheets. Oftentimes, instead of keeping the traditional follow-up note, even of the problem oriented type noted above, a more suitable method is the forming of a graph or flow sheet (Figure 13.7 and 13.8). This flow sheet can be arranged again in the four parts required for "SOAP", but done graphically so an entire hospital stay (or for an outpatient, a year's care) may be visible on a single page. Judicious use of such prospective graphs combined with follow-up notes, can keep the chart from being overly long (a possibility with the problem oriented record).

VI. Patient Summary. If patient is to be transferred, such

Figure 13.7

FLOW SHEET

Date - 1971	Feb 1	15	Mar 1	June 2	Sept 3	Dec 3
200 Headaches	┼┼┼┼	┼┼	—	—	—	—
180 Blood Pressure						
160 Systolic □						
120 Diastolic △						
100 Pulse o						
80 Blood Sugar, 2 hrs. p.c. x						
60						
Ortho Novum	+	—	—	—	—	—
Instructions Diabetes			+			+
Urine Testing				+		
Feet Care					+	
GTT			+			
RX						
RX						

FLOW SHEET
CHEMICAL DIABETES

\#_____

NAME_____

Figure 13.8

FLOW - SHEET

as admission or discharge from hospital, or referral to another physician, a <u>summary</u> should be prepared, listing each problem and the essential data concerning it.

PATIENT SUMMARY

Dear Dr. X:

Mrs. Y. is moving to your town and has asked me to send you a summary of her care. She had the following problems: (1) Headaches, (2) Hypertension, (3) Hyperglycemia, (4) Situational Reaction.

Problem No. 1: Headaches
Onset 6 months ago, on awakening. Negative exam except BP up. Had been on birth control pills since 2 months before headaches started. On discontinuance of birth control pills, headaches disappeared. Patient given size 70 coil spring diaphragm. No Rx given for headaches.

Problem No. 2: Hypertension
Known since 1 February 71. Highest 194/120. Present 120/78. Subsided with discontinuance of anovulatory Rx. No medication needed.

Problem No. 3: Hyperglycemia
1 February 71, 2 hour p.c. blood sugar 164. On stopping anovulatory pills, blood sugar 2 hours p.c. 110, but GTT abnormal, returning to normal 3 hours. Placed on mod CHO restriction.

Problem No. 4: Situational Reaction
Mrs. Y. was born and raised in our rural community. Her husband has done well with the local branch of the tractor company and promotion requires his transfer to the home office. Mrs. Y. is torn between leaving her family and friends and holding back her husband's advancement. She is concerned over her ability to adjust to your big city and will need psychological support. You may, therefore, wish to give her an early appointment.

Final Diagnosis: Iatrogenic headaches and hypertension from anovulatory pills. Chemical Diabetes Mellitus. Situational Reaction.

VII. Discussion. In young people there are fewer problems,
     and all may be related. Older populations often have
     many problems and the inter-relationships are more
     obscure. However, problem orientation serves these
     complicated charts well. An excellent way to follow
     the patient in this example would be to prospectively
     prepare a graphic chart, or flow sheet as illustrated.
     Perhaps a whole year's record could be followed at a
     glance (Figures 13.7 and 13.8).

VIII.Family Records. It might be well to consider from the
     outset having family records rather than only individual
     patient records. This could well consist of an outer
     folder with room for family problems and their solu-
     tions. Place within that outer folder, individual
     folders for each member of the family. One method of
     doing this would be to use vertical filing with edge
     filing of the family number folders. Folders are
     available with tabs for edge filing, including terminal
     digit filing. Then use the ordinary top tabbed folders
     for the individual members of the family. These indi-
     vidual charts could then be numbered with the family
     number followed by an additional digit to indicate the
     family member. Most certainly one should include, in
     the family folder, a problem list as its first page,
     as well as a family data base. The family history might

include such items as financial problems, illness that affects the entire family (such as a crippled father unable to work fulltime, or a mother with rheumatic heart disease which makes her unable to attend to all of her responsibilities, or a severely and chronically ill child that causes family finances or other adjustments to be disturbed). Other family problems might be those of inheritable illnesses such as sickle cell trait. Problems extracted from that data base should be placed on the Problem List and handled similarly to the individual members. Plans should be formulated and stated in the chart for those problems that can be handled on a family basis such as having the "Family Service" arrange for a home helper. Finally, follow-up notes as indicated for the family might well be made and structured quite similarly to the usual POMR follow-up notes.

In summary, a good medical record should start with a complete and up-to-date Problem List on page 1, based on an adequate data base. Plans and follow-up notes are related to specific problems and are structured effectively.

Keep medical records as if "the patient's life depended on them". It may!

Figure 13.1
OUTLINE OF PAST MEDICAL HISTORY

Family History: Cancer - T.B. - Diabetes - Heart Disease -
High Blood Pressure - Strokes - Anemia - Bleeders - Jaundice
Gout - Kidney Disease or Stones - Allergy - Epilepsy -
Longevity - Migraine - Mental Retardation - Consanguinity -
Birth Defects

Marital History: Spouse - Children - G-P-A - Complications
of Pregnancy

Social History: Place of birth - Present home - Travel -
Military Service - Education - Employment - Disability -
Insurance rejection - Exercise - Working hours - Meals -
Appetite - Weight changes - Changes in way of life: Causes -
Tobacco - Alcohol - (Psychedelic) drugs - Medicine

Past History: Immunization - Boosters - Skin tests -
Allergies: Hay Fever - Asthma - Exzema - Hives - Reactions
to medicines - Shots - Transfusions - Bee stings

Previous Illness: Cancer - Tropical Diseases - Rubella -
Mononucleosis - Rheumatic fever - Chorea - Scarlatina -
Venereal disease - Poliomyelitis - Typhoid fever

Previous Injuries: Fractures - Operations - Other Hospita-
lizations

System Review: Headaches - Unconsciousness - Seizures -
Vertigo - Head Injuries

EENT: Poor vision - Infections - Pain - Injuries - Glaucoma
Double vision - Color vision - Hearing - Infection - Injury -
Aches - Tinnitus - Nasal bleeding - Discharge - Sneezing -
Bleeding - Colds - Anosmia - Sore throat - Hoarseness - Sores
or lumps - Lips or tongue - Mouth - Bleeding gums - Dental
problems - Swollen glands or lumps in neck - X-ray Rx to
neck - Difficult or painful swallowing

Cardio-Respiratory: Dyspnea - PND - Orthopnea - Cough -
Night cough - Sputum - Hemoptysis - Fever - Night sweats -
Noisy breathing - Chest pain - Edema - Claudication - Reynaud
Night cramps - Has, or had contact with T.B. - Bronchitis -
Pneumonia - Fungal disease - X-rays or EKG's - Heart attacks
or trouble - High blood pressure, Rx - Varicose veins

Gastro-Intestinal: Indigestion - Abdominal distress - N & V -
Hematemesis - Constipation - Diarrhea - Abnormal stools -
Melena - Bleeding - Hemorrhoids - Jaundice - Hepatitis -

X-rays - Parasites - Ulcers - Cirrhosis - GB Series - Pan-
creatitis

Genito-Urinary: Nocturia - Frequency - Dysuria - Urine color -
Hesitancy - Urgency - Dribbling - Incontinence - V.D. -
Prostatitis - Infection - Retention - Libido - Potentia

Menstrual History: Menarche - Regularity - Timing and duration - Flow - Clots - Cramps - Premenstrual symptoms - Hormone "pills" - Spotting - Discharge - Pruritis - Pain -
Prolapse - Surgery - Hot flashes - Sterility - Overweight
babies - Toxemia - Pap smears - Sex problems

Musculo-Skeletal: Neck ache - Backache - Osteomyelitis -
Joint stiffness - Soreness - Swelling - Leg cramps - Muscle
soreness - Atrophy - Stiffness - Bursitis

Neuro-Psychiatric: Paralysis - Ataxia - Tremor - Stroke -
Tics - Emotional problems - Insomnia - Depression - Anxiety -
Hallucinations

Dermatology: Rashes - Pruritis - Sores - Lumps - Abnormal
tightness - Dark moles

Breasts: Tumors - Nipple discharge - Enlargement - Tenderness

Endocrine: Salt craving - Warmth - Coldness - Polydipsia -
Diabetes - Enlarged head, feet, hands - Goiter - Hair growth
or loss

Hematology: Enlarged nodes - Abnormal blood count - Bleeding -
Purpura

Figure 13.2
PHYSICAL EXAMINATION OUTLINE

VITAL SIGNS:

T____ P____ R____: (RA)____/____, (LA)____/____

BP: (Thigh) _____

Ht._____Wt._____(Ideal)_____Sex_____

Abnormality of pulse_____

GENERAL APPEARANCE: Nourishment - Development - Apparent
age - Alertness - Orientation - Memory - Respiration -
Apparent acute distress

HEAD: Shape - Tenderness (including sinuses) - Bruits or
other abnormalities

EYES: Ophthalmoscopic - Discs - Vessels - Microaneurysms -
Fovea - Wrinkling

ENT: Ears - Tympanic membranes - Mastoid processes - Hearing
Nasal discharge - Blocking - Septal deviation - Polyps

MOUTH: Lips - Tongue - Breath odor - Palate - Uvula -
Pharynx - Tonsils - Teeth and gums

NECK: Rigidity - Limited motion - Carotid palpability -
Equality - Bruits - Venous distension - Masses - Nodes -
Tracheal deviation - Thyroid abnormality

SPINE & BACK: Deformity - Tenderness - Limited motion -
Costovertebral tenderness

CHEST & BREASTS: Configurations - Symmetry - Respiratory
movements - Breasts: Masses - Tenderness - Abnormal discharge

LUNGS: Inspection - Respiratory movements - Fremitus -
Resonance - Diaphragm motion - Breath sounds - Rales -
Rhonchi - Wheezes - Rubs - Vocal resonance - Expiratory
delay - Air flow velocity (match tests)

HEART: Size - Sounds - Gallops - Rub - Murmurs - Radiation -
Rhythm - Other abnormalities

ABDOMEN: Surgical scars - Distension - Venous dilation -
Signs of obstruction - Bowel sounds - Bruits - Organomegally -
Masses - Tenderness - Muscle spasm - Pulsations - Ascites

EXTREMITIES: Joint tenderness, motion, swelling, rubor, deformity - Pulses - Edema - Clubbing - Cyanosis - Varicosities

NEUROLOGICAL: Cranial nerves - Muscle strength - Atrophy - Fasciculations - Coordination - Sensation - Reflexes

GENITALIA: Female: Vulva and vagina - Inflammation - Discharge - Tumors - Clitoral enlargement - Caruncle - Glands - Atrophy - Introitus - Relaxations - Uterus: Prolapse - Size - Position - Mobility - Shape - Consistency - Tumors - Cervix: Patulousness - Firmness - Erosion - Cysts - Tenderness (on motion) - Adnexa: Size - Tenderness - Male: Circumcision - Size - Hernia - Varicocele - Tenderness - Masses

RECTAL: Hemorrhoids - Fissures - Masses - Abnormal stool - Blood - Test for occult blood - Proctosigmoidoscopic exam - Prostate: Size - Consistency - Nodules - Secretions

SKIN: Hair texture and distribution - Skin color - Eruptions - Tumors - Nails

LYMPH NODES: Size - Discreteness - Tenderness

REFERENCES

1. Bjorn, Cross: Problem Oriented Practice. New York, McGraw-Hill, 1970

2. Brodman, K., et al: The Cornell medical index: An adjunct to medical interview. JAMA 140:530, 1949

3. Hurst, Walker: The Problem-Oriented System. New York, Medcom Inc., 1972

4. Kanner IF: Programmed medical history-taking with or without a computer. JAMA 207:317, 1969

5. Kanner IF: The programmed physical examination with or without a computer. JAMA 215:1281, 1971

6. Weed LL: Medical Records, Medical Education, and Patient Care. Cleveland, Case Western Reserve University Press, 1969

7. Yarnall, Wakefield: Acquisition of the History Database. Second edition. Medical Computer Services Association, 1972

CHAPTER 14

The Unwanted Patient

NAOMI BAUMSLAG,
RALPH E. YODAIKEN and HARLEY GORDON

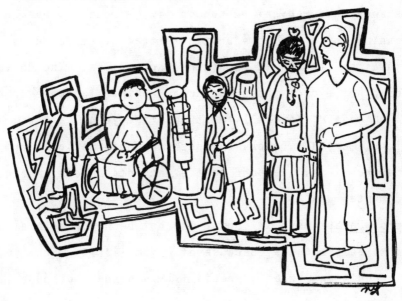

THERE ARE SOME patients unwanted by some doctors,
and others unwanted by most doctors; but whether
they are wanted or not, the doctor must learn to deal with
the patients and himself. The doctor has the right to re-
fuse to treat a patient under his care only if he gives the
patient adequate time to get another physician or if other
arrangements are made for the patient. The decision should
not be hasty. The patient may be unwanted because the problem

is with the doctor or patient or due to circumstances.[21]

Incompatibility: The doctor must try to recognize his own prejudices. Too often the blame is laid at the patient's door if he does not measure up to the doctor's expectations or demands. Very often "the poor" are expected to maintain a standard of medical responsibility - routine physicals, immunizations, health education - that every doctor's family maintains although it is often inaccessible. The doctor should not expect those who speak another language or dialect or who have different life styles (the young, Blacks, Appalachians, Mexicans, etc.) to understand his medical terminology or expressions. Respond to the patient's needs in a non-judgmental way.

Doctor Uneasiness: A doctor may not be happy with a patient who makes him uneasy because of unfamiliarity with the medical condition. When a specialist is needed, discuss it with the patient and help him make the necessary arrangements. Referral is not an excuse for ignorance, and many patients are shunted to specialists unnecessarily. The doctor should be able to treat gonorrhea, provide contraceptive advice and do a PAP smear as part of an annual physical examination or employ allied health personnel who can assist in these areas.

Handicapped Doctor: Sometimes the limitations apply equally to all and are the reflections of limitations of knowledge or of mortality. The doctor may be as much a victim of the

era of "miracles" and rising expectations as the patient.
He should not deny a patient the right to hope. He should
protect him from trying unjustified dangerous, mutilating
or ruinously expensive attempts at treatment.

Night Calls: It is not uncommon for a doctor to be asked
by a patient for emergency care "because I can't disturb my
own doctor at night." The doctor will fulfill his responsibility if he makes adequate arrangements to cover his practice and lets his patients know this.

Fees and Freedom of Choice: The physician is entitled to a
fee for his services and should not be embarrassed to discuss costs and payment with his patients. The patient who
cannot afford the doctor's reasonable fee may be resented.
The inadequately insured patient may also be resented. Increasingly patients are forced to go to a particular doctor
because their choice is limited as in charity hospitals,
health clinics or small towns, and the patient may resent
this. Doctors practicing in institutions or prisons, for
instance, are often viewed as part of the oppressive personnel.

Difficult Patient: The patient may reach the doctor with a
chip on his shoulder because of impersonal attention, long
waits, or fragmented care. The doctor may bear the brunt
of this even though he is not responsible. The disorganized
patient who cannot keep or remember appointments, the panicky
or demanding patient, the patient who medicates himself or

demands medication which is unnecessary and ineffective
(maybe even harmful) are generally unwanted patients, but
their difficulty can be minimized as they get to know and
respect the doctor.

Peripatetic Patient: This patient may have seen many doctors, received multiple diagnoses and had an awe-inspiring
number of pills prescribed for him. It is possible that the
patient may truly be a "difficult" patient. He could, however, be one who is insecure or suffering from the fact that
he attends institutions where no provision is made for continuity of care. No single step will help more than drawing
up a "problem oriented record" and cutting down the therapy
to justified and manageable proportions. Occasionally the
doctor may have difficulty in convincing the patient that
therapy mindlessly renewed from year to year is not necessary. Recently a patient was seen who had been put on a
3 week trial of anti-convulsants for "restlessness". The
therapy stretched on for 10 years and he was only persuaded
to stop it with great difficulty. The patient is free to
accept or reject advice. If the doctor feels that the rejection of advice is detrimental to the patient, he should
discuss the reasons for the regime or routine with the patient and try to find out the reasons for noncompliance.

Informed (Misinformed?) Patient: The patient may be able
to give the doctor a great deal of accurate information.

The doctor should not resent the fact or feel challenged.
When one of us (H.G.) saw his first case of familial dysau-
tonia, diagnosed elsewhere, the patient's father was able
to inform him about the disease and its management.   His
experience was invaluable and the leaflets produced by a
group of parents of similar patients was extremely informative.   However, the patient also may be misinformed.   The doctor should remember that news reports, radio and television
announcements, drug house claims and eccentrics may supply
inaccurate information.   In addition, the doctor himself may
find it impossible to know whether he is in favor of widely
publicized measures such as multiphasic screening, whether
PAP smears are really worthwhile, whether radical is better than simple mastectomy and so on.   In remembering that
yesterday's medical orthodoxy is sometimes today's quackery,
he will sympathize with the patient who avidly hopes that
the medical profession can find answers to all problems.

SPECIAL CONSIDERATIONS

   Mechanization of our society has enabled technical skills
to be applied in many areas such as heart valves and pace-
makers for cardiac patients, intracerebral valves and shunts
for children with meningoceles or spina bifida, limbs for
amputees and a variety of appliances for otherwise deformed
and handicapped children and adults.   Those who used to die
at birth or at an early age are now kept alive.[10]   Parents are

called on to deal with emotional problems, mechanical gadgets
medication and social restrictions.[2,9,10,13]

The physically and mentally handicapped, the addict,
the attempted suicides, the teenage mothers and the alcoholics
are a large segment of our society. As physicians, we have
to devote our efforts not only to short term medical problems
and grateful patients but also to chronically ill and sometimes seemingly ungrateful patients. The attempts which
have been made to put away some of these neglected people
has resulted in the development of ugly institutions which
are poorly run, costly and a drain on the resources of the
individual, the family and the state.

Condemned to Life: The cessation of extraordinary and expensive measures for prolonging life unnecessarily and uselessly
may be needed for patients with partially remediable but
ultimately lethal defects; with disseminated malignancy; or
who are kept artificially alive on respirators or venous and
arterial catheters. The doctor has to remember that the
quality of life granted a patient is an important consideration and so is the viewpoint of the family.[15] Many legal
hassles have occurred where the doctor has "done things" for
the patient without consulting the family.[6]

Handicapped Patients: The handicapped child and the family
require intelligent support. In order to assure the family
and avoid fragmentation under stress, the physician has to

be aware of the anxieties and anticipate future problems
such as schools, social interactions, occupation and, if
possible, marriage. Sex and love cannot be denied to people
just because they are handicapped.[16] They have a right to
love. The physician has to recognize the possibility that
the family with which he is dealing may have to live outside
the normal and accepted social environment. Therefore, this
family is in constant need of reassurance as well as advice.
Assuring a "normal and productive life" for the physically
handicapped is a cliche if in the process the family unit
disintegrates under the strain. The physician who undertakes
the care of such patients must not only be readily available
for consultation with respect to medication, but also has to
be a general counselor, suggesting ways and means of easing
the financial burden such as legitimate tax "write-offs" or
directing the breadwinner to a tax consultant; and suggesting
church groups, neighbors or locally concerned agencies that
may be able to advise the family about physical or social
relief. Advice on what "should be done" is lip service
unless practical suggestions are included. It is preferable
to visit, call or write to the agency that helps the handicapped. Frequently, these agencies are only able to supply
literature and token advice. Financial aid and other practical methods of assistance are more difficult to obtain.
Some agencies are very specific about the financial groups

to whom they offer aid, and a modest income can turn out
to be an insurmountable obstacle to a family in need of a
wheel-chair.

The Free Clinic Patient: The role of the medical practitioner as an adviser is important in many areas, but it is
not his prerogative to pass judgment, and advice should not
be confused with judgment. It is probably the moral judg-
mental practice of some practitioners that has led to the
opening of "free clinics" where medical advice is available
from doctors who are sympathetic and understanding rather
than superior and moralistic. An unmarried teenager who
requests birth control pills or even an abortion should be
told where to seek competent help rather than given a lecture
on morals.[8,22] Advice on the use of contraceptive techniques
and the various indications and contraindications to such
techniques are practical measures which are the stock and
trade of the free clinics. A trustworthy friend may be the
most important part of the cure. Usually an alcoholic or
drug addict who has been through this "scene" and is now
cured is the best friend to a similarly afflicted person.
Addicted Patient:[3,5,17] The alcoholic suffers nutritional
problems, peripheral neuropathy, hepatic, pancreatic and
myocardial disease as well as being more susceptible to infection and trauma. Deprived of alcohol, he may function;
supplied with it, he does not. Drug addiction is a far less

important, although much more publicized, public health
problem. The drug addict given his drug, functions; deprived
of it, he does not. The health problems associated with the
drug addict depend on the drug used. Heroin is the most important addicting drug, both because of the publicity accorded
the problem and the social consequences of its illegality.
The heroin addict may be poorly nourished as well as susceptible to infection or hepatitis from contaminated syringes,
and subject to imprisonment or injury. He may be forced to
resort to prostitution. In the United States heroin main-
tenance is frowned on, but Methadone treatment is accepted.
The addict is often intelligent and plausible and will continue to importune the doctor for drugs as long as the doctor
accedes to his request. Also the addict admitted to a hospital or the patient who seeks relief of withdrawal should
be given substitution drugs to control the withdrawal. Group
therapy and psychiatric help is often of value. The treatment of addiction is unlikely in the absence of the patient's
strong wish to be cured. Attesting to this is the comparative success of Alcoholics Anonymous and the drug free therapeutic communities. It is hoped that society will one day,
in the absence of a better solution, allow the addict his
drugs.

The Endocrine Patient: The ugliest of all patients are the
organically ill whose disease is unsuspected; the recalcitrant

truculent patient with an insulinoma and bouts of hypoglycemia; the hirsute, garulous adrenal cortical adenoma; the
peculiar eccentric hypercalcemic with a parathyroid adenoma;
the dour, good for nothing myxedema; and the hysterical Grave
disease. How many organically ill and potentially curable
patients are housed in instutitions for the insane is anyone's guess. They make up the unaccounted number of patients
who are put out of sight because their symptoms mask the
signs and it may be far less trouble to institutionalize them
than to diagnose their problem.

On the other hand, the disease may take years to manifest and may, in fact, for the life span of the patient be
a "slow burner" giving rise to endless family misery unre-
lieved by the paliative therapy given by the doctor. Many
of these patients may never be sufficiently ill to require
hospitalization. We have seen a sufficient number of patients of this type treated for years as nuisances, to wish
that every outpatient clinic and private waiting room had a
neon sign, "Doctor! Are you sure your Unwanted Patient is
not an endocrine disorder?"

The Aged Patient:[4,11]   The problems of the aged are often
related to an increasing dependency on others. Everyone
loves a baby - few love an old man or an old woman. The
elderly often suffer from cataracts, glaucoma, diabetes,
arteriosclerosis, and mental deterioration. Visual and

auditory acuity may be diminished. They need motivation and
activity - a purpose in life. The mental problem may be real
but not infrequently, it is the result of some deficiency
disease such as vitamin B_{12}, folate or iron deficiency which
are all common in this age group. Trauma is poorly tolerated,
and recovery from even slight incapacitation is slow. To
provide meaningful help to an elderly patient requires evaluation of that individual's state of independence in terms of
speech, vision, hearing, the ability to manage finances, to
shop and walk. The elderly may be mentally alert, creative
and aware of current issues or they may be bedridden, unable
to dress, or cook for themselves. Each person has to be
assessed as an individual and not as a group although, ultimately, the individual may well be introduced to a group with
whom he or she can identify.

The Dying Patient:[12,14,20] In other cultures and less techno-
logical societies, death is familiar and accepted. In our
society the dying are segregated and death rejected. At what
point a patient is a dying patient depends on our and his
appreciation of the fact. Those familiar with "primitive"
people recognize the dying person's ability to accept death
and die peacefully - to decide to die. In the past, ordinary
people have been familiar with how to deal with death, and
artists have recognized the mechanisms dying people adopt
to cope with death. Few case histories could equal the

description of Prince Andrey's death in <u>War and Peace</u>.[19] Doctors ought to know how to cope with death, so that the dying
patient doesn't find himself alone and uncomforted, in a
conspiracy of silence. The patient, knowing he is dying,
is forced to join this conspiracy of silence out of respect
for his doctor's and relatives' feelings. This unrealistic
approach to death also leaves the relatives ill prepared for
grieving. The patient should be given the opportunity to
put his affairs in order and die in familiar surroundings.[7]

. . . .

Although many problems in society affect health, the
solution of these problems is not to be accomplished by
medical care alone. The doctor cannot fill the void left
by the disappearance of the older generation from the family,
the loneliness which results from the mobility of Americans,
and the loss of committment to religion which has resulted
in the loss of the minister as a family counselor. Never-
theless, the doctor will frequently find himself cast in
this role - particularly in a society which believes there
is a meaning to life and will strive to work with others to
improve the system.

REFERENCES

1. Calland CH: Iatrogenic problems in end stage renal failure. New Eng J Med 287:334, 1972

2. Care of the mentally subnormal. Lancet 2:727, 1969 (Editorial)

3. Criteria Committee, National Council on Alcoholism: Criteria for the diagnosis of alcoholism. Amer J Psychiat 129:127, 1972

4. DiCicco L, Apple DA: Health needs and opinions of older adults. Sociological Studies in Health and Sickness. Edited by DA Apple. New York, McGraw Hill, 1966

5. Drug Abuse. Report to Ford Foundation. New York, Praeger Publishers, 1972

6. Epstein LC, Lasagna L: Obtaining informed consent: Form or substance. Arch Intern Med 123:682, 1969

7. Fletcher J: The patient's right to die. Harpers 221: 139, 1960

8. Furstenberg F, Gordis L, Markowitz M: Birth control knowledge and attitudes among unmarried pregnant adolescents: A preliminary report. J Marriage and Family 31:34, 1969

9. Grossman FK: Brothers and Sisters of Retarded Children. Syracuse, Syracuse University Press, 1972

10. Intensive care and low birth-weight. Lancet 2:1183, 1972 (Editorial)

11. Isaacs B: Geriatric patients: Do their families care? Br Med J 4:282, 1971

12. Kubler-Ross E: On Death and Dying. New York, MacMillan, 1970

13. Mather HG, Pearson NG, Read KLQ: Acute myocardial in- farction: Home and hospital treatment. Br Med J 3: 334, 1971

14. Mitcheson R: A surgeon's duty. Br Med J 1:186, 1965 (Letter)

15. Rickham, Johnston: Neonatal Surgery. New York,
    Appleton, Century, Crofts, 1969

16. A Right to Love? Lancet 1:1057, 1972 (Editorial)

17. Sapira JD: The narcotic addict as a medical patient.
    Amer J Med 45:555, 1968

18. Shaw GB: The Doctor's Dilemma, Getting Married, and
    The Shewing-Up of Blanco Posnet. New York, Brentano's,
    1911

19. Tolstoy L: War and Peace. Translated by L Maude.
    New York, Simon & Schuster, 1942

20. Verwoerdt A: Communication with the Fatally Ill.
    Springfield, Chas C. Thomas, 1966

21. Von Mering O: Value dilemmas and reciprocally evolved
    transactions of patient and curer. Psychoanalyst 49:
    119, 1962

22. Waters JL: Pregnancy in young adolescents: A syndrome
    of failure. Southern Med J 62:655, 1969

Abbreviations

This list of abbreviations is available to standardize the contractions used so that not only will you understand what is written, but so that it provides permanent decipherable documentation of "facts". Try to use the abbreviations provided and if you come across others, add them to the list.

A$_2$	aortic valve second sound
AAL	anterior axillary line
AB	abortion
abd.	abdomen
AC	alternating current; anterior chamber (eye)
A.C.	Alcoholic Clinic
a.c.	before meals
AC & BC	air conduction and bone conduction (of ear)
acid p'tase	acid phosphatase
ACTH	andrenocorticotropic hormone
A.D.	right ear (Latin: auris dextra)
A.D.C.	Aid to Dependent Children (Welfare)
A.F.A.	Aid for the Aged (Welfare)
AFB	acid fast bacilli (usually mycobacteria)
AGN	acute glomerulonephritis
A/G	albumin/globulin
A.H.F.,A.H.G.	anti-hemophilic factor; anti-hemophilic globulin
A.I.	aortic regurgitation
AJ	ankle jerk
ALA	amino levulinic acid
ALL	acute lymphoblastic leukemia
a.m.a.	against medical advice (signing out of hospital)
AML	acute myeloblastic leukemia

AMML	acute myelomonoblastic leukemia
AP	abdonimo-perineal
A-P	anteroposterior
A & P	auscultation and percussion
A-P & Lat.	anteroposterior and lateral
APB	atrial premature beat
APC	atrial premature contraction; aspirin-phenacetin-caffeine
ARF	acute rheumatic fever
AS	arteriosclerosis
A.S.	aortic stenosis; left ear (Latin: auris sinistra)
A.S.A.	acetylsalicylic acid (aspirin)
at. fib.	auricular fibrillation
A.T. 10	dehydrotachysterol
A-V	arteriovenous
a. & w.	alive and well
baso., bas.	basophil
B_1C	beta-1-C globulin, part of complement system
BCP	birth control pills
BCS	battered child syndrome
BDC	brain damaged child
B.E.	barium enema
b.f.	bottle fed; breast fed
b.i.d.	twice a day (Latin: bis in die)
BIH	bilateral inguinal hernias

bisp.	bispinous or intraspinous diameter
bili.	bilirubin
B.J.	biceps jerk
b.m.	bowel movement; bone marrow; blood and mucus
B.M.R.	basal metabolic rate
BOMA	bilateral otitis media, acute
B.O.W.	bag of waters (aminon and its fluid)
B.P.	blood pressure
B.P.H.	benign prostatic hypertrophy
B.P.S.	bilateral partial salpingectomy
b.s.	bowel sounds; breath sounds
BSP	bromsulphalein (a liver function test)
BT	bleeding time
BUN	blood urea nitrogen, regulated by glomerular filtration rate
bx	biopsy
$\bar{c}$	with (Latin: cum)
C_1, C_2	first cervical vertebra, second, etc.
Ca	calcium
CA	carcinoma or cancer
cap.	capsule
cath	catheter
CBC	complete blood count
c.c.	chest circumference, chronic cervicitis
C.C.	Central Clinic

CC	Chief Complaint
cc.	cubic centimeter
C.C.T.	chocolate coated tablet
CCU	Coronary Care Unit
ceph. floc.	cephalin flocculation test
CGH	chorionic gonadotropin hormone
CGN	chronic glomerular nephritis
CHD	congenital heart disease, coronary heart disease
CHF	congestive heart failure
chr.	chronic
C.I.D.	cytomegalic inclusion disease
Cl	chloride
cldy.	cloudy
CLL	chronic lymphocytic leukemia
cm.	centimeter
CMC	chloramphenicol (Chloromycetin)
CML	chronic myelocytic leukemia
CNS	central nervous system
c/o	complaining of
CO_2	carbon dioxide
cont.	continued
C.P.	cerebral palsy
CPC	clinicopathological conference; Central Psychiatric Clinic
CRP	C reactive protein

C and S	culture and sensitivity (for bacteria)
c.s.f.	cerebrospinal fluid
CSR	corrected (erythrocyte) sedimentation rate
c.t.	clotting time
C.V.A.	cerebrovascular accident
CVD	cardiovascular disease
DA	drug addict
DC	diagonal conjugate
D & C	dilation and curretage
D_1, D_2	first thoracic (dorsal vertebra), second, etc.
d/c, D.C.	discontinue
decr.	diminished or decreased
Derm.	Dermatology
diag.	diagnosis
diag. conj.	diagonal conjugate (a pelvic measurement
diff.	differential white count
disch.	discharge
Disp.	disposition
DLE	disseminated lupus erythematosus
DOA	dead on arrival
DOE	dyspnea on exertion
D.P.T.	diphtheria, pertussis, tetanus immunization
D.T.D.	give of such a dose (Latin: datur talis dosis)

D.T.'s	delirium tremens
DTR's	deep tendon reflexes
D & V	diarrhea and vomiting
DVT	deep vein thrombosis
D5W	5% dextrose in water solution
dx	diagnosis
ECD	exposure to contagious disease
ECG	Electrocardiogram (EKG may be preferred for legibility)
ECHO virus	enteric cytophathogenic human orphan viruses
E.C.T.	electroconvulsive therapy; enteric coated tablet
ecz.	eczema
E.D.C., or E.D.D.	estimated date of confinement (or delivery)
EEG	electroencephalogram
EKG	electrocardiogram
ENT	ear, nose and throat
EOM	extraocular movements
E.O.M.	Emergency Operating Room
E.R., E.W.	emergency room, emergency ward
ESR	erythrocyte sedimentation rate
exp.	expiration or expiratory
F.	Flatus
fam. doc.	family doctor
fam. phys.	family physician

FB	foreign body
FBS	fasting blood sugar
FH	Family History
FHR	fetal heart rate
f.h.s.	fetal heart sounds
FHT	fetal heart tones
fib.	fibrillation
flut.	flutter
for. body	foreign body
frac.; fx.	fracture
freq.	frequent
FTLEFV (LOA)	full term, low elective forceps; vertex presentation (see fetal position)
FTNLCM	full term normal living colored male
F/U	follow-up
g.b.	gall bladder
g.c.	gonorrhea, gonoccus
GE	gastroenteritis
G.I.	gastrointestinal
GI or Grav. I	primigravida, secundigravida, etc.
gluc.	glucose
GPD	glucose 6-phosphate dehydrogenase
Gm.	gram
Gm. %	grams per hundred milliters of serum
G.O.E.	nitrous oxide (gas), oxygen, ether anesthesia

Gold So.	colloidal gold curve
gr.	grain
Grav. II, etc.	indicating a woman of so many pregnancies regardless of outcome
GSW	gunshot wound
GTT	glucose tolerance test
GU	genitourinary
Gyn	Gynecology
H.C.	head circumference
Hct.	hematocrit
H.C.V.D.	hypertensive cardiovascular disease
H.C.G.	human chorionic gonadotropin
HEENT	head, eyes, ears, nose, throat
Hgb., Hb.	hemoglobin
H-J reflux	Hepato-jugular reflux
HMD	hyaline membrane disease
H.O.	House Officer
H.P.F.	high power (microscope) field
h.s.	bed time (Latin: hora somni)
ht.	height
hypt.	hypertension
I.C.S.	intercostal space
ICU	Intensive Care Unit
IDM	infant of diabetic mother
I & D	incision and drainage

I.E.P.A.	immunoelectrophoresis
I.H.	infectious hepatitis
IM	intramuscular
Imp.	impression
incr.	increased or increasing
insp.	inspiration or inspiratory
IPPB	intermittent positive pressure breathing
I.Q.	intelligence quotient
IT	inter-tuberous
ITP	idiopathic thrombocytopenic purpura
I.U.	international units
I.U.D.	intra-uterine device
IUP	intro-uterine pregnancy
131_I	radioactive iodine
ITP	idiopathic thrombocytopenic purpura
IVP	intravenous pyelogram
JRA	juvenile rheumatoid arthritis
J.V.D.	jugular venous distension
K	potassium
Kg.	kilogram
k.j.	knee jerk
KUB	kidney, ureter, bladder (x-ray - plain film of abdomen)
L	left
L_1, L_2	first lumbar vertebrae, second, etc.
L & A	light and accommodation

lab.	laboratory
LAP	leukocyte alkaline phosphatase
lat.	lateral
lb.	pound
LBBB	left bundle branch block (of cardiac conduction)
LBCD	left border of cardiac dullness
LDH	lactic dehydrogenase
L.E.	lupus erythematosus
L.F.	liver failure
LFA	left frontoanterior
LFP	left frontoposterior
LFT	left frontotransverse
L.K.S.	liver, kidney, spleen
LLL	left lower lobe (lung)
LLQ	left lower quadrant (abdomen)
LMA	left mentoanterior
LMD	local medical doctor
LMLE	left medio-lateral episiotomy
LMP	last menstrual period, left mento-posterior
LMT	left mentotransverse
LNMP	last normal menstrual period
LNN	lower nephron nephrosis
LOA	left occiput anterior
LOP	left occiput posterior

LOT	left occiput transverse
L.P.	lumbar puncture
L.P.N.	Licensed Practical Nurse
LSB	left sternal border
LTCS	low transverse caesarian section
LUL	left upper lobe (lung)
LUQ	left upper quadrant (abdomen)
LVH	left ventricular hypertrophy
l. & w.	living and well
lymphs	lymphocytes
lytes	electrolytes
m	murmur
M_1	mitral first sound
MA	mental age, megaloblastic anemia
MAL	mid axillary line
MC	mental confusion
mcg.	microgram
MCH	mean corpuscular hemoglobin
MCHC	mean corpuscular hemoglobin concentration
MCL	mid clavicular line
MCV	mean corpuscular volume
m.d.	manic depressive
meds.	medications
mEq (meq/L)	milliequivalents (per liter)
M.H.B.	maximum hospital benefit

mg.	milligram
Mg	magnesium
mg%	milligrams per hundred milliliters of serum of blood
M.I.	myocardial infarction, mitral insufficiency
ml.	milliliter (s) (preferred over cc.)
MLE	midline episiotomy
mm. Hg.	millimeters of mercury (blood pressure)
MOM	milk of magnesia
MMM	myelofibrosis with myeloid metaplasia
mono.	monocyte, mononucleosis
M.R.	mental retardation
M.T.D.	right ear drum (membrane tympanidextra)
M.T.S.	left ear drum (membrane tympanisinistra)
N	nocturia
Na	sodium
N/A	not applicable
NDAR	no diagnostic abnormalities recognized
N.D.R.	neurotic depressive reaction
Neuro, or neuro	Neurology or neurological
NG	naso-gastric
NGUD	no genitourinary disease
nl.	normal
NPH	neo-protamine Hagedorn (long acting insulin)
NPN	non-protein nitrogen (see BUN)

NPO	nothing by mouth (Latin: Nihil per os)
NR	not remarkable, normal
NSP	non-specific prostatitis
NSU	non-specific urethritis
O_2	oxygen
O_2 cap.	oxygen capacity
O_2 sat.	oxygen saturation
O.B.S.	organic brain syndrome
o.c.	obsessive compulsive
O.C.	obstetrical conjugate
Occ.	occasional
Occ. Th.	Occupational Therapy
O.D.	right eye (Latin: oculus dexter), overdue
Op.	operation
O.P.D.	Out-Patient Department
OPV	oral polio vaccine
OR	operating room
oriented x 4	oriented to time, place, person and situation
O.S.	right eye (Latin: oculus sinister)
OT	old tuberculin
O.U.	both eyes or either eye
P.	pulse
P_2	pulmonic second heart sound
P.A.	pernicious anemia

P-A	posteroanterior
PAC	premature atrial contraction
PAL	posterior axillary line
P.A.P.	cytologic test for cancer first described by Papanicolaou
para	number of infants born alive
Para I or P.I., Para II, etc.	primipara, secundipara, etc. indicating a woman with so many births regardless of neonatal death
P.A.T.	paroxysmal atrial tachycardia
Pb	lead
PBI	protein bound iodine
p.c.	after meals (Latin: post cibum)
pcn	penicillin
PCO_2	partial pressure carbon dioxide
P.D.R.	Physician's Desk Reference
PE	physical examination
Ped.	Pediatric
P.E.P.	protein electrophoresis
Percuss & ausc. (P & A)	percussion and auscultation
PERRLA	pupils equal, round and react to light and accommodation
pH	hydrogen ion concentration
PH, PMH	Past History, Past Medical History
PHLA	post-heparin lipolytic activity
p.m.	post mortem examination
p.i.d.	pelvic inflammatory disease (salpingitis)

P.K.U.	phenylketonuria
P.M.I.	point of maximum impulse (of heart)
PMP	previous menstrual period
P.N.C.	Prenatal Clinic
p.n.d.	paroxysmal nocturnal dyspnea, postnatal drip
PO_2	partial pressure oxygen
PO_4	phosphorus
p.o.	post operative; by mouth (Latin: per os)
polys	polymorphonuclear leucocytes
poplit.	popliteal
post	post-mortem examination
PPBS	postprandial blood sugar
p.p.d.	purified protein derivative (for tuber-culin test)
PPP	polyuria, polydipsia, polyphagia
P.R.	pityriasis rosea
p.r.	per rectum
prem.	premature
prep.	prepare
p.r.n.	as often as necessary (Latin: pro re nata)
PROM	premature rupture of membranes
pro. T., pro time	prothrombin time
p-s	psychosomatic
PSP	phenolsulfonphthalein (excretion test of renal function)

pt.	patient
P.T.	Physical Therapy
p.t.a.	prior to admission
P.T.T.	partial thromboplastin time, prothrombin time
PZI	protamine zinc insulin (long acting insulin)
PV	per vagina (pelvic)

Pelvic Measurement

Ant. (or) Post Sag. D.	anterior (or) posterior sagittal diameter
A-O D	anterior diameter
bisp.	bispinous or interspinous diameter
DC	diagonal conjugate
IT	intertuberous
OC	obstetrical conjugate
Trans. D.	transverse diameter
q.	every
q. 2h	every two hours
q.d.	daily (Latin: quaque die)
q.h.	every hour (Latin: quaque hora)
q.h.s.	every night at bedtime
q.i.d.	four times per day (9 a.m., 1 p.m., 5 p.m., 9 p.m. at CGH)
q.m.	every morning
q.o.d.	every other day
R	right

R., resp.	respiration
RAI	radioactive iodine
RBBB	right bundle branch block
RBC	red blood count
rbc	red blood cell
RBOW	ruptured bag of waters (amniotic rupture)
ref. doc.	referring doctor
R.E.S.	reticuloendothelial system
RF	renal failure
RFA	right frontoanterior
RFP	right frontoposterior
RFT	right frontotransverse
RFX	refractory
Rh	Rhesus blood factor
RHD, RF	rheumatic heart disease, rheumatic fever
R.J.	radial reflex jerk
RLQ	right lower quadrant
RMA	right mentoanterior
RMP	right mentoposterior
RMT	right mentrotransverse
R.N.	Registered Nurse
R/O	rule out
RSA	right sacrum anterior
RSP	right sacrum posterior

RST	right sacrum transverse
RTC	return to clinic
RUQ	right upper quadrant
R_x	therapy, treatment
$\bar{s}$	without (Latin: sine)
S_1, S_2	first sacral vertebra; second, etc; also first and second heart sounds
S_3	ventricular gallop
S_4	atrial gallop
SAP	serum alkaline phosphatase
S.B.	stillborn
SBE	subacute bacterial endocarditis
SC prep	sickle cell preparation
sed. rate	sedimentation rate
SGOT	serum glutamic oxalacetic transaminase
SGPT	serum glutamic pyruvic transaminase
SH	Social History, serum hepatitis
sig.	label (Latin: statim)
sl.	slight
stat	at once (Latin: statim)
S.M.W.	social medical worker
S.M.W.D.Sep.	single, married, widowed, divorced, separated
S.O.B.	short of breath
S.O.S.	if necessary (Latin: si opus sit)
S.M.R.	submucous resection

sp. gr., S.G.	specific gravity
S.R.	schizophrenic reaction
ss.	a half (Latin: semis)
T.	temperature
T_1, T_2	first thoracic vertebra, second, etc.
T_3	tri-iodothyronine
T_4	thyroxine
T & A	tonsillectomy and adenoidectomy
T.B., tbc.	tuberculosis
tbsp.	tablespoon
T & C	type and crossmatch (blood for transfusion)
Tc	technetium, most commonly used radionuclide for imaging
T.C.	Therapeutic Community
tcn.	Tetracycline
T-G	triglycerides
t.i.d.	three times a day (9 a.m., 3 p.m., 9 p.m.)
TIFD	tissue insufficient for diagnosis
TINEM	there is no evidence of malignancy
TINEN	there is no evidence of neoplasm
TL	tubal ligation
TLC	tender loving care
t.m.	tympanic membrane
TPR	temperature, pulse, respiration
tr., tinct.	tincture

tsp.	teaspoon
T.T.	thrombin time
T.U.R.	transurethral resection
Tx	treatment
UCG	urine chorionic gonadotropin
UCHD	usual childhood diseases
ULQ	upper left quadrant
umb.	umbilical
ung.	ointment
URI	upper respiratory infection
urt.	urticaria
UTI	urinary tract infection
VD	venereal disease
VDRL	serologic test for syphilis (venereal disease research laboratory)
VMA	vanillyl mandelic acid
VU	varicose ulcer
V. tac.	ventricular tachycardia
WBC	white blood cell count
WDWN	well-developed well nourished
wks. gestat.	weeks gestation
WNL	within normal limits
x	times; power

Selected Bibliography

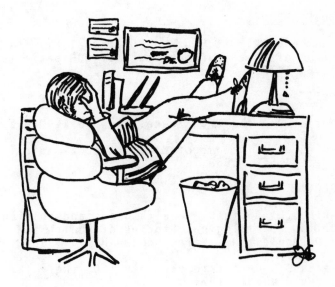

ABDOMINAL PAIN

Rang EH, Fairbairn AS, Acheson ED: An inquiry into the incidence and prognosis of undiagnosed abdominal pain treated in hospitals. Br J Prev Soc Med 24:47, 1970

ACCURACY

Garland LH: Studies of the accuracy of diagnostic procedures. Amer J Roentgen 82:25, 1959

ACUTE ABDOMEN

Staniland JR, Ditchburn J, De Dombal FT: Clinical presentation of acute abdomen study of 600 patients. Br Med J 3:393, 1972

ADDICT

Louria DB: The Drug Scene. New York, McGraw-Hill, 1968

Sapira JD: The narcotic addict as a medical patient. Amer J Med 45:555, 1968

AGED

DiCicco L, Apple D: Health needs and opinions of older adults. Sociological Studies of Health and Sickness. Edited by DA Apple. New York, McGraw-Hill, 1960

Isaacs B: Geriatric patients: Do their families care? Br Med J 4:282, 1971

Tips on how and where to manage that elderly patient. Patient Care 3:86, 1969 (Editorial)

Williams EI, Bennett FM, Nixon JV, et al: Sociomedical study of patients over 75 in general practice. Br Med J 2:445, 1972

ALCOHOL

Bales RF: Cultural differences in rates of alcoholism. Sociological Studies of Health and Sickness. Edited by DA Apple. New York, McGraw-Hill, 1960

Edwards G: Patients with drinking problems. Br Med J 4:435, 1968

Szasz TS: Bad habits are not diseases. Lancet 2:83, 1972

ALLERGY

Drug allergy: Therapeutic conference. Br Med J 2:37, 1971

ALLIED HEALTH (see MANPOWER)

AMBULATORY CARE

Bellinin SS, Geiger HJ, Gibson CD: Impact of ambulatory
health care services on the demand for hospital beds. New
Eng J Med 280:808, 1969

Lewis CE, Resnik BA, Schmidt G, et al: Activities, events
and outcomes in ambulatory patient care. New Eng J Med 280:
645, 1969

Lewis CE, Resnik BA: Relative orientations of students of
medicine and nursing to ambulatory patient care. J Med
Educ 41:161, 1966

Nigro SA: A psychiatrist's experiences in general practice
in a hospital emergency room. JAMA 214:1657, 1970

Organization of ambulatory care. Ambulatory Pediatrics.
Edited by M Green, RJ Haggerty. Philadelphia, W.B. Saunders
Co., 1968

AMNIOCENTESIS

Edwards JH: Uses of amniocentesis. Lancet 1:608, 1970

ANENCEPHALY AND SPINA BIFIDA

Naggan L, MacMahon B: Ethnic differences in the prevalence
of anencephaly and spina bifida in Boston, Massachusetts.
New Eng J Med 277:1119, 1967

ANTIBODIES

Antibodies against tumours. Br Med J 4:505, 1971 (Editorial)

ASTHMA

Assessment and management of severe asthma. Lancet 1:1055,
1972 (Editorial)

Knapp PH: The asthmatic and his environment. J Nerv Ment
Dis 149:133, 1969

ATOPIC

Rhyne MB: The atopic disorders.   Ambulatory Pediatrics.
Edited by M Green, RJ Haggerty.   Philadelphia, W.B. Saunders
Co., 1968

ATTITUDES (also see SOCIO-CULTURAL)

Aring CD: In respect of youth.   Arch Intern Med 124:383,
1969

Crosby DL, Waters WE: Survey of attitudes of hospital staff
to cadaveric kidney transplantation.   Br Med J 4:346, 1972

Furstenberg F, Gordis L, Markowitz M: Birth control knowledge and attitudes among unmarried pregnant adolescents:
A preliminary report.   J Marriage Family 31:34, 1969

Jacoby NM: Unrestricted visiting in a children's ward.
Lancet 2:584, 1969

Kegeles SS: Attitudes and behavior of the public regarding
cervical cytology: Current findings and new directions for
research.   J Chronic Dis 20:911, 1967

Kurtz R, Hoffning R: Attitudes toward the lower and middle
class psychiatric patient as a function of authoritarianism
among mental health students.   J Consult Clin Psychol 35:
338, 1970

McMahon AW, Shore MF: Some psychological reactions to
working with the poor.   Arch Gen Psychiat 18:563, 1968

Redlich FC, Hollingshead AB, Bellis E: Social class dif-
ferences in attitudes toward psychiatry.   Sociological
Studies of Health and Sickness: A Source Book for the
Health Professions.   Edited by D Apple.   New York, McGraw-
Hill, 1960

Wigfield AS: Attitudes to venereal disease in a permissive
society.   Br Med J 4:342, 1971

Willie C: The social class of patients that public health
nurses prefer to serve.   Amer J Public Health 50:1126, 1960

AUTISM

Greenfeld J: A Child Called Noah.   New York, Holt, Rinehart
and Winston, 1972

BACK PAIN

Freyberg RH: Back pain. Signs and Symptoms: Applied Pathologic Physiology and Clinical Interpretation. Edited by CM MacBryde, RS Blacklow. Philadelphia, J.B. Lippincott Co., 1970

BATTERED CHILD

Gill D: Violence Against Children. Cambridge, Harvard University Press, 1970

Jackson G: Child abuse syndrome: The cases we miss. Br Med J 2:756, 1972

Kempe CH, Helfer RE: Helping the Battered Child and His Family. Philadelphia, Lippincott Co., 1972

BEHAVIOR

Berne E: Transactional Analysis in Psychotherapy. New York, Grove Press, 1970

Dubos R: So Human an Animal. New York, Charles Scribner's and Sons, 1968

Harris TA: I'm Okay, You're Okay: A Practical Guide to Transactional Analysis. New York, Harper and Row, 1969

Knutson AL: The Individual, Society and Health Behavior. New York, Russell Sage Foundation, 1965

McKeown T, Lowe C: Modification of personal behavior. Introduction to Social Medicine. Philadelphia, F.A. Davis Co., 1966

Pond MA: Interpersonal relations in medical settings. Public Health Rep 76:967, 1961

Rutter M, Tizard J, Whitmore TK: Education, Health and Behavior. London, Longman Co., 1970

Walsh J, Elling R: Professionalism and the poor: Structural effects and professional behavior. J Health Soc Behav 9:16, 1968

BIRTH CONTROL

Contraceptives-Current status of therapy. JAMA 214:2316, 1970 (Editorial)

Furstenberg F, Gordis L, Markowitz M: Birth control knowledge and attitudes among unmarried pregnant adolescents:
A preliminary report. J Marriage Family 31:34, 1969

BIRTH DEFECTS

National Association for Mental Health Working Party: Birth
of an abnormal child: Telling the parents. Lancet 2:1075,
1971

Nelson MM, Forfar JO: Associations between drugs administered during pregnancy and congenital abnormalities of the
fetus. Br Med J 1:523, 1971

BRAIN DAMAGE

Towben A: Organic causes of minimal brain dysfunction.
JAMA 217:1207, 1971

BREAST FEEDING

Jelliffe DB, Jelliffe EFP: The uniqueness of human milk.
Amer J Clin Nutr 24:970, 1971 (Symposium)

Pryor K: Nursing Your Baby. New York, Harper and Row, 1963

BURNS

Andreasen NJC, Noyes R, Hartford CE: Management of emotional
reactions in seriously burned adults. New Eng J Med 286:
65, 1972

Martin HL, Lawrie JH, Wilkinson AW: The family of the
fatally burned child. Lancet 2:628, 1968

CHILD ABUSE (see BATTERED CHILD)

CHILDBIRTH

Bradley RA: Husband-Coached Childbirth. New York, Harper
and Row, 1965

Dick-Read G: Childbirth without Fear. Second edition.
New York, Harper and Row, 1960

CHILD CARE

Childrearing: Its Social and Psychological Aspects. Edited
by SA Richardson, AF Guttmacher. Baltimore, Williams and
Wilkins Co., 1967

Connor BH: Mothers and infants in the Transkei. Lancet 1: 768, 1968

Court SDM: Child health in a changing community. Br Med J 2:125, 1971

Deprivation of Maternal Care: A Reassessment of its Effects. Edited by MD Ainsworth. Geneva, World Health Organization, WHO Public Health Pap No 14, p. 165, 1962

How the Scots feed their babies. Lancet 1:403, 1968 (Editorial)

Leavitt SR, Gofman H, Harvin D: Uses of developmental charts in teaching well child care. Pediatrics 31:499, 1963

Life in flats. Br Med J 1:661, 1970 (Editorial)

Plight of one-parent families. Br Med J 2:667, 1972 (Editorial)

Williams CD, Jelliffe DB: Mother and Child Health: Delivering the Services. New York, Oxford University Press, 1972

CHRONIC DISEASE

Bennett AE, Garrad J, Halil T: Chronic disease and disability in the community: A prevalence study. Br Med J 3:762, 1970

Mattson A: Long-term physical illness in childhood: A challenge to psycho-social adaptation. Pediatrics 50:801, 1972

COLDS

Mortimer EA: Frequent colds. Ambulatory Pediatrics. Edited by M Green, RJ Haggerty. Philadelphia, W.B. Saunders Co., 1968

COMMUNICATION (also see DOCTORS & PATIENTS)

Bates RC: The Fine Art of Understanding Patients. Oradell, Medical Economics, 1968

Blum LH: Reading between the Lines. New York, International University Press, 1972

Boyl CM: Differences between patients and doctors interpretation of some common medical terms. Br Med J 2:247, 1970

Cartwright A: Patients and Their Doctors: A Study of General Practice. New York, Atherton Press, 1967

Cochrane AL, et al: Observer errors in taking medical histories. Lancet 1:1007, 1951

Croog S: Interpersonal relations in medical settings. Handbook of Medical Sociology. Edited by HE Freeman, S Levine, LG Reeder. Englewood Cliffs, Prentice Hall Inc., 1963

Egbert LD: Reduction of postoperative pain by encouragement and instructions to patients. New Eng J Med 270:825, 1964

Epstein LC, Lasagna L: Obtaining informed consent: Form or substance. Arch Intern Med 123:682, 1969

Frances V, Korsch BM, Morris MJ: Gaps in the doctor-patient communication. New Eng J Med 280:535, 1969

General knowledge of cancer. Br Med J 4:381, 1972 (Editorial)

A guide to understanding teenagers. Patient Care 1:22, 1967 (Editorial)

Informed (but uneducated) consent. New Eng J Med 287:465, 1972 (Editorial)

Kahn JH: Communication with children and parents. Br Med J 3:406, 1972

Korsch BM, Negrete VF: Doctor-patient communication. Sci Amer 227:66, 1972

Ley P, Spelman MS: Communication with Patient. Lancet 1: 663, 1970

Meares A: Communication with the patient. Lancet 1:663, 1970

Rogers CR, Stevens B: Person to Person: The Problem of Being Human. Lafayette, Real People Press, 1967

Verwoerdt A: Communication with the Fatally Ill. Springfield, Chas. C. Thomas, 1966

Von Mering O: Value dilemmas and reciprocally evolved transactions of patient and curer. Psychoanalyst 49:119, 1962

COMMUNITY CARE (also see HEALTH CARE)

Are young people's ills clues to community ills? Public
Health Rep 84:198, 1969

Burgess R, McKegney EP: The community health visitor program: A student organized experiment. J Med Educ 44:193,
1969

Court SDM: Child health in a changing community. Br Med
J 2:125, 1971

Goodrich CH, Olendzki M, Deuschle KW: Mount Sinai's approach
to the East Harlem community. Bull NY Acad Med 46:97, 1970

Haggerty RJ: Problems of teaching comprehensive community
care. Amer J Dis Child 116:509, 1968

Lewis CE, Easton R: Community medicine: Personality characteristics, career interests, observed health behavior and
teaching. Arch Environ Health 21:99, 1970

Logan RFL: Assessment of sickness and health in the community: Needs and methods. Med Care 2:173, part 2:218, 1964

Paxton H: Community medicine unites town and gown. Hospital
Physician 6:68, 1970

Wallace HM, et al: The role of physicians trained in maternal and child health in community service and teaching: A
follow-up report. Pediatrics 42:512, 1968

CONGENITAL DEFECTS (see BIRTH DEFECTS)

CONGENITAL HEART DISEASE

Perloff JK: The Clinical Recognition of Congenital Heart
Disease. Philadelphia, W.B. Saunders Co., 1970

CONGENITAL HIP

Congenital dislocation of the hip. Br Med J 2:6, 1971
(Editorial)

CONSUMER PROTECTION (see ETHICS)

COUGH

Gregg RH: Cough. Ambulatory Pediatrics. Edited by M
Green, RJ Haggerty. Philadelphia, W.B. Saunders, 1968

CULTURE (see SOCIO-CULTURAL)

CYSTIC FIBROSIS

McCollum AT, Gibson LE: Family adaptation to the child with cystic fibrosis. J Pediat 77:571, 1970

CYTOLOGY

Kegeles SS: Attitudes and behavior of the public regarding cervical cytology: Current findings and new directions for research. J Chronic Dis 20:911, 1967

Saneran E: Cytology screening. Error Rate in Cytology Automation. Edited by DM Evans. Edinburgh, Livingstone Ltd., 1970

DEATH

Care of the dying. Lancet 2:753, 1971 (Editorial)

Early deaths. Br Med J 4:315, 1971 (Editorial)

Fletcher J: The patient's right to die. Harpers 221:139, 1960

Goldfarb AI: Death and Dying: Attitudes of Patient and Doctor. New York, Group for the Advancement of Psychiatry, 1965

Kennell JH, Slyter H, Klaus MH: The mourning response of parents to the death of a newborn infant. New Eng J Med 283:344, 1970

Kozol J: Death at an Early Age. New York, Bantam, 1970

Kubler-Ross E: On Death and Dying. New York, MacMillan, 1970

The paradox of death and the "omnipotent" family doctor. Patient Care 4:14, 1970 (Editorial)

Sudden deaths in infants. Lancet 2:1070, 1971 (Editorial)

DENTAL CARE

Burket: Oral Medicine. Sixth edition. Philadelphia, Lippincott and Co., 1971

Kriesberg L, Treiman B: Dentists and the practice of dentistry as viewed by the public. J Amer Dent Ass 64:806,
1962

Lambert C, Freeman H: The Clinic Habit. New Haven, College
and University Press, 1967

DEVELOPMENT

Brazelton TB: Infants and Mothers: Individual Differences
in Development. New York, Seymour Lawrence, 1969

Illingworth RS: Development of the Infant and Young Child,
Normal and Abnormal. London, Livingstone Ltd., 1970

Leavitt R, Gofman H, Harvin D: Use of developmental charts.
Pediatrics 31:499, 1963

DIABETES

Baumslag N, Yodaiken RE, Varady J: Standardization of
terminology in diabetes types and family history. Diabetes
119:664, 1970

Diabetes mellitus: Disease or syndrome. Lancet 1:583,
1971 (Editorial)

Edwards JH: Should diabetics marry? Lancet 1:1045, 1969

DIET

Crosby WH: Iron enrichment: One's food, another's poison.
Arch Intern Med 126:911, 1970

Edwards CH, McSwain H, Haire S: Odd dietary practices of
women. J Amer Diet Ass 30:976, 1954

Simoons FJ: Eat Not This Flesh. Madison, University of
Wisconsin Press, 1961

DISABILITY

Types of Injuries: Incidence and Associated Disability.
N.C.H.S. U.S. Dept H.E.W., Series 10, No. 57, 1969

DOCTORS & PATIENTS (also see COMMUNICATION)

Balint: The Doctor, His Patient, His Illness. New York,
International Universities Press Inc., 1972

Blackgell B: When do physicians expect their patients to come to them. Med Care 7:155, 1969

Jaco EG: Patients, Physicians and Illness. New York, Free Press, 1958

Jones RO: How to avoid making your patient sicker. Consultant 10:10, 1970

Truman S: The Doctor, His Career, His Business, His Human Relations. Baltimore, Williams and Wilkins Co., 1951

DOGMA

Beazley JM, Underhill RA: The fallacy of the fundal height. Br Med J 4:404, 1970

Blishen B: Doctors and Doctrines. Toronto, University of Toronto Press, 1969

Bolande RP: Ritualistic surgery - circumcision and tonsillectomy. New Eng J Med 280:591, 1969

Dann TC: Routine skin preparation before injection. Lancet 2:96, 1969

Haggard P: Devils, Drugs and Doctors. New York, Simon and Schuster, 1959

Surgical rituals. Br Med J 3:543, 1972 (Editorial)

DRUGS

Freestone DS: Formulation and therapeutic efficacy of drugs used in clinical trials. Lancet 2:98. 1969

Koch-Weser J: Serum drug concentrations as therapeutic guides. New Eng J Med 287:227, 1972

Lasagna L: 1938-1968 - the FDA, the drug industry, the medical profession and the public. Safeguarding the Public. Edited by J Blake. Baltimore, John Hopkins University Press, 1970

Lennard HL, et al: Hazards implicit in prescribing psychoactive drugs. Science 169:438, 1970

Nelson MM, Forfar JO: Associations between drugs administered during pregnancy and congenital abnormalities of the fetus. Br Med J 1:523, 1971

Nithman CJ, Parkhurst YE, Sommers EB: Physicians   prescribing
habits. JAMA 217:585, 1971

Pillard RC: Marihuana. New Eng J Med 283:294, 1970

Sapira JD: The narcotic addict as a medical patient. Amer
J Med 45:555, 1968

ECONOMICS

Darley W, Somers AR: Medicine, money and manpower: The
challenge to professional education, No. II. New Eng J Med
276:1291, 1967

Eiler RD: National health insurance: What kind and how
much (second of two parts). New Eng J Med 284:945, 1971

Erlich JL: Breaking the dole barrier: The lingering death
of the American welfare system. Social Work 14:49, 1969

Ginzberg E, Ostow M: Men, Money and Medicine. New York,
Columbia University Press, 1970

McNerney WJ: Why does hospital care cost so much? New Eng
J Med 127:76, 1971

Rayack E: Professional Power and American Medicine: The
Economics of the AMA. New York, World Publishing Co., 1967

EDUCATION (also see MEDICAL EDUCATION)

Rutter M, Tizard J, Whitmore TK: Education, Health and
Behavior. London: Longman Co., 1970

EMOTIONAL PROBLEMS

Haldane JD: Emotional problems of childhood and adolescence:
How to use child psychiatry. Br Med J 3:520, 1972

ENURESIS

Meadow R: Childhood enuresis. Br Med J 4:787, 1970

ENVIRONMENT

Bregman, Jacob I: Man, water and environment. Arch Environ
Health 20:100, 1970

Hunter D: The Diseases of Occupations. Fourth edition.
Boston, Little, Brown and Co., 1969

Rosen S: Noise hearing and the cardiovascular function.
The Physiological Effects of Noise. Edited by Welch, Welch.
New York, Plenum Press, 1970

EPIDEMIOLOGY

Pike MC, Morrow RH: Statistical analysis of patient control:
Studies in epidemiology. Br J Prev Soc Med 24:42, 1970

EPILEPSY

Supplementary treatment of epilepsy. JAMA 214:1973, 1970
(Editorial)

ETHICS

Human research. New Eng J Med 286:372, 1972 (Editorial)

Lappe M, Gustafson JM, Roblin R: Ethical and social issues
in screening for genetic disease. New Eng J Med 286:1129,
1972

Ramsey P: The Patient as Person: Explorations in Medical
Ethics. New Haven, Yale University Press, 1970

Torrey EF: Ethical Issues in Medicine: The Role of the
Physician in Today's Society. Boston, Little, Brown and
Co., 1968

Zachary RB, Leeds MB: Ethical and social aspects of treatment of spina bifida. Lancet 2:274, 1968

EXPERIMENTATION

Jonas H: Philosophical reflections on experimenting with
human subjects. Daedalus 98:219, 1969

FAMILY

Billingsley A: Family functioning in the low-income black
community. Social Casework 50:563, 1969

Binger CM, et al: Childhood leukemia: Emotional impact on
patient and family. New Eng J Med 280:414, 1969

Debushey M: The Chronically Ill Child and His Family.
Springfield, Charles C. Thomas, 1970

Elliot K: The Family and Its Future. Ciba Foundation Symposium. London, J & A Churchill, 1970

Family Use of Health Services U.S. 1963-1964. N.C.H.S.
U.S. Public Health Service Publications, Series 10, No. 55,
1969

Group for the Advancement of Psychiatry: The Case History
Method in the Study of Family Process, VII, 76. New York,
GAP Publishing Office, 1970

Group for the Advancement of Psychiatry: The Field of
Family Therapy VII, 78. New York, GAP Publishing Office,
1970

Handicapped children and family stress. Br Med J 1:329,
1972 (Editorial)

Hill: Social stresses on the family. Social Casework 39:
139, 1958

Hurell GD, Sturdy P, Frood JDL: Viruses in families.
Lancet 1:769, 1971

Incest and family disorder. Br Med J 2:364, 1972 (Editorial)

Laing RD, Esterson A: Sanity, Madness and the Family:
Families of Schizophrenics. New York, Basica Books, 1965

Martin HL, Lawrie JH, Wilkinson AW: The family of the
fatally burned child. Lancet 2:628, 1968

Matsen JM, Turner JA: Reinfection in enterobiasis (pinworm
infection): Simultaneous treatment of family members.
Amer J Dis Child 118:575, 1969

McCollum AT, Gibson LE: Family adaptation to the child
with cystic fibrosis. J Pediat 77:571, 1970

McKinney GE: Adapting family therapy to multi-deficient
families. Social Casework 51:327, 1970

Mead M, Heyman K: The Family. New York, Macmillan Co.,
1965

Meyer RJ, Haggerty RJ: Streptococcal infections in families -
factors altering individual susceptibility. Pediatrics 29:
539, 1962

Olsen SH: The impact of serious illness on the family
system. Postgrad Med 47:169, 1970

Selected Family Characteristics and Health Measures. N.C.H.S
U.S. Dept. HEW, Series 3, No. 7, 1967

Stein Z: The families of dull children: A classification
for predicting careers. Br J Prev Soc Med 14:83, 1960

FAMILY PRACTICE (also see HEALTH CARE and MANPOWER)

Beloff GS, Weinerman ER: Yale studies in family health care
I. Planning and pilot tests of a new program. JAMA 199:383,
1967

Beloff GS, Snoke P, Weinerman ER: Yale studies in family
health care II. Organization of a comprehensive family care
program. JAMA 204:355, 1968

Bower AD: Medical care: Its social and organizational
aspects (general practice - an analysis and some suggestions).
New Eng J Med 269:667, 1963

Geyman JP: The Modern Family Doctor and Changing Medical
Practice. New York, Appleton-Century-Crofts, 1971

Group for the Advancement of Psychiatry: The Field of
Family Therapy. Report No. 78, GAP Reports and Symposiums
7:519, 1970

Haggerty RJ: Etiology and decline in general practice.
JAMA 185: 179, 1963

Lees DS, Cooper MH: The work of the general practitioner.
J Coll Gen Practice 6:408, 1963

McFarlane AH, O'Connell BP: Morbidity in family practice.
Canad Med Ass J 101:259, 1969

Roemer MI: General physician services under eight national
patterns. Amer J Public Health 60:1893, 1970

Villaveces JW, Welcher WH, Evans GR: A family practice
survey in Ventura County. Calif Med 117:85, 1972

Walton HJ: The psychiatric component in general practice.
Lancet 2:35, 1970

Zabarenko L, Zwell ME: Training for Family Practice: A
Selected Bibliography. Pittsburgh, University of Pittsburgh,
1970

FORGOTTEN PATIENTS

The forgotten. Br Med J No. 5749-5756, 1971
    I.   A paralyzed man. p. 603
    II.   A woman with epilepsy. p. 661
    III.   A single woman. p. 721
    IV.   Motor neurone disease. p. 40
    V.   A man with multiple sclerosis. p. 102
    VI.   The unmarried mother. p. 162
    VII.   A family. p. 215
    VIII. An occupation centre. p. 272

GASTROENTERITIS

Matthew TS: Infantile gastroenteritis. Br Med J 3:161, 1970

GENETIC (also see COUNSELING)

Edwards JH: Uses of amniocentesis. Lancet 1:608, 1970

Genetic Counseling. Br Med J 1:458, 1972 (Editorial)

Gordan H: Genetic counseling. JAMA 217:1215, 1971

Leonard CO, Chase GA, Childs B: Genetic counseling: A consumer's view. New Eng J Med 287:433, 1972

Raine DN: Management of inherited metabolic disease. Br Med J 2:329, 1972

The pregnancy at risk for a genetic disorder. New Eng J Med 282:627, 1970 (Editorial)

Yen S, MacMahon B: Genetics of anencephaly and spina bifida. Lancet 2:623, 1968

GESTATION

Length of gestation. Br Med J 4:582, 1970 (Editorial)

HANDICAPPED

Allen RC: Legal Rights of the Disabled and Disadvantaged. Washington, D.C., U.S. Dept HEW, Superintendent of Documents, U.S. Govt. Printing Office

Aspects of handicap. Lancet 1:113, 1972 (Editorial)

Baumslag N, Yodaiken RE: Care of "special people". New
Eng J Med 286:1220, 1972 (Letter)

Handicapped children. Br Med J 3:179, 1970 (Editorial)

Hospital services for the mentally ill. Lancet 2:1368,
1971 (Editorial)

HEADACHE

Wolf HG: Headache. Signs and Symptoms: Applied Pathologic
Physiology and Clinical Interpretation. Edited by CM
MacBryde, RS Blacklow. Philadelphia, Lippincott Co., 1970

HEALTH CARE (also see MANPOWER)

The administrator meets the consumer. Medical Opinion and
Review 6:18, 1970

Alpert J: Broken appointments. Pediatrics 34:127, 1964

Alpert J: Slave patients and free physicians. New Eng J
Med 284:667, 1971

Anderson RA: A Behavioral Model of Families' Use of Health
Services Research Studies, #25. Center for Health Administration Studies, the University of Chicago, 1968

Bates JE, et al: Provisions for health care in the ghetto:
The family health team. Amer J Public Health 60:1222, 1970

Baumann B: Diversities in conception of health and physical
fitness. J Health Hum Behav 2:39, 1961

Bergan SS, Schatzki M: New directions for an urban hospital.
JAMA 215:935, 1971

Bryant J: Health and the Developing World. Ithaca, Cornell
University Press, 1970

Can community centers cure health problems of the poor?
JAMA 211:943, 1970 (Editorial)

Chaney E, et al: How well do patients take oral penicillin:
Collaborative study in private practice. Pediatrics 40:
188, 1967

Cohen WJ: Current problems in health care. New Eng J Med
281:193, 1969

Conference Proceedings: The Role of Maternal and Child
Health and Crippled Children's Programs in Evolving Systems
of Health Care. The University of Michigan Medical Center.
Ann Arbor: The University of Michigan, 1970

Coser R: Life in the Ward. E. Lansing, Michigan State
University Press, 1962

Coughey JL: Education of the physician for his role in comprehensive health service. J Med Educ 34:581, 1959

Curran WJ: The "class-action" approach to protecting health
care - consumers - the right to psychiatric treatment. New
Eng J Med 286:26, 1972

Darley W, Somers AR: Medicine, money and manpower - the
challenge to professional education, No I. New Eng J Med
276:1234, 1967

Darley W, Somers AR: Medicine, money and manpower - the
challenge to professional education, No. III. New Eng J
Med 276:1414, 1967

Darley W, Somers AR: Medicine, money and manpower - the
challenge to professional education, No. IV. New Eng J Med
276:1471, 1967

Elsom KO: Elements of the medical process. JAMA 217:1216,
1971

Engel GL: A unified concept of health and disease. Perspect
Biol Med 3:459, 1960

Fraser DM: Congress, the physician and health planning.
Medical Opinion and Review 6:27, 1970

Friedson E: Client control and medical practice. Amer J
Sociol 65:374, 1960

Fuchs VR: The growing demand for medical care. New Eng J
Med 279:190, 1968

Gales H: The community health education project bridging
the gap. Amer J Public Health 60:322, 1970

Griffith HW: Instructions for Patients. Philadelphia,
W.B. Saunders Co., 1968

Gubner RS: Changes in the physician's role in health care:
Causes and effects. Ann NY Acad Sci 166:832, 1969

Haggerty RJ: The academic health center and health care delivery: Preparing personnel to meet the demand. J Med Educ 46:3, 1971

Haggerty RJ: The boundaries of health care. Pharos 35:106, 1972

Heagarty M, Robertson LS: Slave doctors and free doctors - a participant observer study of the physician-patient relation in a low-income comprehensive care program. New Eng J Med 284:636, 1971

Lee RV: Provisions of health services - past, present and future. New Eng J Med 277:682, 1967

Lepper MH: Health planning for the urban community. Public Welfare 25:141, 1967

Lerner R, Kirchner C: Social and economic characteristics of municipal hospital outpatients. Amer J Public Health 56:884, 1966

Magraw RM: Ferment in Medicine: A Study of the Essence of Medical Practice and Its New Dilemma. Philadelphia, W.B. Saunders Co., 1966

Marston RW: To meet the nation's health needs. New Eng J Med 279:520, 1968

Mather HG, Pearson NG, Read KLQ: Acute myocardial infarction: Home and hospital treatment. Br Med J 3:334, 1971

McKinlay JB: The new late comers for antenatal care. Br J Prev Soc Med 24:52, 1970

Mechanic D: Public Expectations and Health Care. New York, Wiley-Interscience, 1972

Medical Care in Developing Countries: A Symposium from Makerere. Edited by M King. Nairobi, Oxford University Press, 1966

Menke WG: The political background of health planning. Medical Opinion and Review 6:32, 1970

Menke WG: Professional values in medical practice. New Eng J Med 280:930, 1969

Millis JS: The future of medicine - the role of the consumer. JAMA 210:501, 1969

Murnaghan JH, White KL: Hospital patient statistics: Problems and prospects. New Eng J Med 284:822, 1971

Mustell RR: Health planning and physician responsibility.
Medical Opinion and Review 6:24, 1970

Palmer DL, Reed WP, Kisch AL: Health in a rival hippie
commune. JAMA 213:1307, 1970

Revans R: Research into hospital management and organization. Milbank Memorial Fund Q 44:No. 3, 1966, Part 2.
Health Services Research I

Richmond JB: Currents in American Medicine. Cambridge,
Harvard University Press, 1969

Somers AR: Who's in charge here? - or Alice searches for a
king in Mediland. New Eng J Med 287:849, 1972

Storey PB, Roth RB: Emergency medical care in the Soviet
Union. JAMA 217, 588, 1971

Thompson GE, Glick SM: Municipal hospital patient care.
Arch Intern Med 127:673, 1970

White KL, Williams TF, Greenberg BG: The ecology of medical
care. New Eng J Med 265:885, 1961

White KL: Primary medical care for families - organization
and evaluation. New Eng J Med 277:847, 1967

Willie C: The social class of patients that public health
nurses prefer to serve. Amer J Public Health 50:1126, 1960

HEALTH EDUCATION

Cobb WM: Health education for disadvantaged youth.   Ann
NY Acad Sci 166:889, 1969

Pellegrino ED: Human values and the medical curriculum.
JAMA 209:1349, 1969

HEARING

Parker W: Hearing and age. Geriatrics 24:151, 1969

HOME CARE

Holt KS: The home care of severely retarded children.
Pediatrics 22:744, 1958

HOME VISITS

Marsh GN, McNay RA, Whewell J: Survey of home visiting by
general practitioners in northeast England. Br Med J 1:487,
1972

HOSPITAL PRACTICE

Ginzberg E, Rogatz P: Planning for Better Hospital Care.
New York, Columbia University Press, 1961

HYPERACTIVE

Stewart MA: Hyperactive children. Sci Amer 222:94, 1970

IATROGENIC

Calland CH: Iatrogenic problems in end-stage renal failure.
New Eng J Med 287:334, 1972

Herbst AL, Ulfelder H, Poskanzer D: Adenocarcinoma of the
vagina: Association with maternal stilbestrol therapy with
tumor appearance in young women. New Eng J Med 284:878, 1971

Hyperkinetic child and stimulant drugs. New Eng J Med 287:
249, 1972 (Editorial)

Nelson MM, Forfar JO: Associations between drugs administered during pregnancy and congenital abnormalities of the
fetus. Br Med J 1:523, 1971

Rowe WS: Iatrogenic disease. Med J Aust 2:560, 1969

Safer D, Allen R, Barr E: Depression of growth in hyperactive children on stimulant drugs. New Eng J Med 287:217,
1972

Stewart AM, Kneale GW: Age distribution of cancers caused
by obstetric x-rays and their relevance to cancer latent
periods. Lancet 2:4, 1970

Todd JW: Errors of medicine. Lancet 1:665, 1970

IMMUNIZATION

For and against smallpox vaccination. Br Med J 2:311, 1970
(Editorial)

Meyer HM, Parkman PD: Rubella vaccination: A review of
practical experience. JAMA 215:613, 1971

Prophylaxis against rubella and mumps. Br Med J 2:282, 1970
(Editorial)

The Report of the Committee on Infectious Diseases. Evanston,
Amer Acad of Pediat, 1972

INFORMED CONSENT (see COMMUNICATION)

INTELLECT

Intellectual Maturity of Children as Measured by the
Goodenough-Harris Drawing Test. N.C.H.S. U.S. Dept. HEW,
Series 11, No. 105, 1970

LEAD POISONING

Chisolm JJ: Poisoning due to heavy metals. Pediat Clin
N Amer 17:591, 1970

Control of Lead Poisoning in Children. U.S. Dept. HEW,
Public Health Service, Bureau of Community Environmental
Management, 1970

Lin-Fu JS: Lead Poisoning in Children. Children's Bureau,
HEW, Pub. #452, Superintendent of Documents, U.S. Govt
Printing Off., 1967

LEARNING DISORDERS

Kappelman MM, Luck E, Ganter RL: Profile of the disadvantaged child with learning disorders. Amer J Dis Child 121:
371, 1971

LOW BIRTH WEIGHT

Intensive care and low birth weight. Lancet 2:1183, 1972
(Editorial)

LOW-INCOME

Alpert JJ, Kosa J, Haggerty RJ: A month of illness and
health care among the low-income families. Public Health
Rep 82:705, 1967

Bergner L, Yerby AS: Low-income and barriers to use of
health services. New Eng J Med 278:541, 1968

Bierman P: Meeting the health needs of low-income families.
Ann Amer Acad Polit Soc Sci 337:103, 1961

Coles R: The doctor and newcomers to the ghetto. The
American Scholar 40:66, 1970-71

DeVise P, et al: Slum Medicine: Chicago's Apartheid.
Health System, Report No. 6 of the Interuniversity Social
Research Committee, Chicago: Community and Family Study
Center, University of Chicago, 1969

Greenblatt EM, Emery PE, Glueck BC: Poverty and Mental
Health. Psychiatric Research Report #21 of the American
Psychiatric Assoc., Washington, D.C., Amer Psy Assoc, 1967

Holloman JLS: Medical care and the black community. Arch
Intern Med 127:51, 1971

McMahon AW, Shore MF: Some psychological reactions to
working with the poor. Arch Gen Psychiat 18:563, 1968

Mental Health of the Poor. Edited by F Riessman, et al.
New York, Free Press, 1964

Norman JC: Medicine in the ghetto. New Eng J Med 281:1271,
1969

Norman JC: Medicine in the Ghetto. New York, Appleton-
Century-Crofts, 1969

Triplett JL: Characteristics and perceptions of low-income
women and use of preventive health services - an exploratory
study. Nurs Res 19:140, 1970

The Urban Condition. Edited by L Duhl. New York, Basic
Books, 1963

Wershow AJ: Pathogenesis of urban slums. JAMA 215:1959,
1971

Yerby A: The problems of medical care for indigent populations. Amer J Public Health 55:1212, 1965

MANPOWER (also see HEALTH CARE)

Bunker JP: Surgical manpower: A comparison of operations
of surgeons in the USA and England and Wales. New Eng J
Med 282:134, 1970

Cauffman JG, et al: Community health aides: How effective
are they? Amer J Public Health 60:1904, 1970

Cromwell FS: Factors affecting personnel utilization. Amer
J Occup Ther 24:541, 1970

Estes EH, Howard DR: Paramedical personnel in the distribution of health care. Arch Intern Med 127: 70, 1971

Fenninger LD: Health manpower, scope of the problem. Ann
NY Acad Sci 166:825, 1969

Greenfield CH, Brown C: Allied Health Manpower: Trends
and Prospects. New York, Columbia University Press, 1969

Hiscoe DB: Nurses in a crossfire. JAMA 212:294, 1970

Kissick WL: Effective utilization: The critical factor in
health manpower. Amer J Public Health 58:23, 1968

Kissick WL: Health manpower in transition. Milbank Mem
Fund Q 46(Supp):53, 1968

Physician's assistants hired by V.A. HSMHA Health Reports
86:331, 1971 (Editorial)

Role of the nurse. Br Med J 3:659, 1970 (Editorial)

Simpson GA: The family health worker at the community field
level. Ann NY Acad Sci 166:916, 1969

Tanner LA, Carmichael LP: The role of the social worker in
family medicine training. J Med Educ 45:859, 1970

Westheimer RK, et al: Use of paraprofessionals to motivate
women to return for postpartum check-up. Public Health
Rep 85:625, 1970

MEASUREMENT

The Kinetics of Growth. Lancet 2:1234, 1970 (Editorial)

To weigh and to consider. Lancet 2:641, 1970 (Editorial)

Widdowson EM: Harmony of growth. Lancet 1:901, 1970

MEDICAL EDUCATION

Baker L: Our ailing medical schools. Saturday Review 53:
56, 1970

Becker H: Boys in White. Chicago, University of Chicago
Press, 1961

Bruess CE: An approach to preparing health majors. J Sch
Health 40:545, 1970

Campbell M, et al: Management education. Hospitals 44:100,
1970

Carnegie Commission on Higher Education: Higher Education
and the Nation's Health: Policies for Medical and Dental
Education. New Jersey, McGraw-Hill, 1970

Cohen WJ: Medical education and physician manpower from
the national level. The New Physician 17:358, 1968

Engstrom WW: Residency training in internal medicine, for
what: Sub-specialty boards, what for? Ann Intern Med 70:
621, 1969

Haggerty RL: Family medicine: A teaching program for medical students and pediatric house officers. J Med Educ 37:
531, 1962

Hogness JR: The responsibility of the academic health
science center to other health education programs in the
community. Ann NY Acad Sci 166:885, 1969

Jeffereys PM: The teaching of community medicine in the
undergraduate curriculum. Br Med J 3:176, 1969

Lewis CE: A study of the effects of a multidisciplinary
home-care teaching program on the attitudes of first year
students. J Med Educ 41:195, 1966

Meyer RJ: Medical education and medical practice demonstra-
tions. J Med Educ 38:596, 1963

Miller S: Prescription for Leadership: Training for the
Medical Elite. Chicago, Aldine Pub. Co., 1970

New curricula and training for patient care. Arch Intern
Med 124:506, 1969 (Editorial)

Parmelee AH, et al: Well baby clinics in the first year
medical curriculum: The family medicine course at the
University of California at Los Angeles. J Med Educ 35:
675, 1960

Slatter C: Student participation in curriculum planning
and evaluation. J Med Educ 44:675, 1969

Walsh J: Medical education and world health. The New
Physician 18:819, 1969

Weed LL: Medical Records, Medical Education and Patient
Care. Chicago, Year Book Medical Publishers, 1969

White KL: Family medicine, academic medicine and the university's responsibility. JAMA 185:192, 1963

Whitman RM, Viney L: The teaching of doers. Arch Gen
Psychiat 24:379, 1971

NEWBORN

Davis J: Immediate problems at birth. Br Med J 4:164, 1971

Dubowitz LMS, Dubowitz V, Goldberg C: The clinical assessment of gestational age in the newborn infant. J. Pediat
77:1, 1970

Infection in the nursery. Br Med J 3:235, 1970 (Editorial)

Low birth weight and intensive care. Br Med J 3:657, 1970
(Editorial)

Storrs CN, Taylor MRH: Transport of sick newborn babies.
Br Med J 3:328, 1970

Vulliamy DG: Less urgent problems and minor abnormalities.
Br Med J 4:547, 1971

NUTRITION

Birch HG: Functional effects of fetal malnutrition. Hospital
Practice 6:134, 1971

Edelstein T, Metz J: Reduction of incidence of prematurity
by folic acid supplementation in pregnancy. Br Med J 1:16,
1970

Gopalan C, Naidu N: Nutrition and fertility. Lancet 2: 1077, 1972

Krueger RH: Some long-term effects of severe malnutrition in early life. Lancet 2:514, 1969

Naeye RL, Diener MM, Dellinger WS, Blanc WA: Urban poverty: Effects on prenatal nutrition. Science 166:1026, 1969

Obesity and Health: A Source Book of Current Information for Professional Health Personnel. U.S. Dept. HEW, P.H.S. Pub. No. 1485

PAGOPHAGIA

Reynolds RD, et al: Pagophagia and iron deficiency anemia. Ann Intern Med 69:435, 1968

PATIENTS & ILLNESS (see DOCTORS & PATIENTS)

PATIENT'S VIEW (also see ATTITUDES and COMMUNICATION)

Freidson E: The Patient's View of Medical Practice. New York, Russell Sage Foundation, 1961

PHOTOSENSITIVITY

Harber LC, Levine CM: Photosensitivity dermatitis from household products. Am Fam Physician 39:95, 1969

PICA

Lanzkowsky P: Investigation into the aetiology and treatment of pica. Arch Dis Child 34:140, 1959

POVERTY (also see LOW-INCOME)

Frantz F: Wretched of the Earth. Translated by C Farrington. New York, Grove Press, Inc., 1968

Leo PA, Rosen G: A bookshelf on poverty and health. Amer J Public Health 59:591, 1969

PREGNANCY

Dangers of iodides in pregnancy. Lancet 1:1273, 1970 (Editorial)

Gordis L, et al: Evaluation of a program for preventing adolescent pregnancy. New Eng J Med 282:1078, 1970

Hibbard BM: Pregnancy diagnosis. Br Med J 1:593, 1971

Mind and childbirth. Br Med J 2:120, 1971 (Editorial)

Robinson R: The pre-term baby. Br Med J 4:416, 1971

Smithells RW, Speidel BD: Prenatal influences and prenatal diagnosis. Br Med J 4:105, 1971

Treatment of bacteriuria in pregnancy. Br Med J 4:631, 1970 (Editorial)

Waters JL: Pregnancy in young adolescents: A syndrome of failure. Southern Med J 62:655, 1969

PREJUDICE

Lennane KJ, Lennane RJ: Alleged psychogenic disorders in women - possible sexual prejudice. New Eng J Med 288:273, 1973

PRIMARY CARE (also see AMBULATORY CARE, HEALTH CARE, TEAM)

Carmichael LP: Who will give primary care? JAMA 215:1662, 1971

Dubos R: Mirage of Health. New York, Doubleday, 1961

Jacobs AR, Garrett JW, Wersinger R: Emergency department utilization in an urban community. JAMA 216:307, 1971

Our Ailing Medical System: It's Time to Operate. Editors of Fortune. New York, Harper & Row, 1970

PSYCHIATRY

Biological Psychiatry, Vol. I. Edited by JH Masserman. New York, Grune & Stratton, Inc., 1959

Gordon JS: Who is mad? Who is sane? Atlantic Monthly 227: 50, 1971

Kadushin C: Why People Go to Psychiatrists. New York, Atherton Press, 1969

Nelsen JC: Treatment of patients with minor psychosomatic disorders. Social Casework 50:581, 1969

Social Psychiatry (Research Publications Association for
Research in Nervous and Mental Disease XLVII). Edited by
FC Redlich. Baltimore, Williams and Wilkins Co., 1969

QUALITY

Gonnella JS, et al: Evaluation of patient care: An approach.
JAMA 214:2040, 1970

Kessner DM, Kalk CE, Singer J: Assessing health quality:
The case for tracers. New Eng J Med 288:189, 1973

Shapiro S: End result measurements of quality medical care.
Milbank Mem Fund Q 45:7, 1967

RECORDS

Chamberlin RW: Social data in evaluation of the pediatric
patient deficits in out-patient records. J Pediat 78:111,
1971

Weed LS: Quality control and the medical record. Arch
Intern Med 127:101, 1971

REHABILITATION

Brewerton DA, Daniel JW: Factors influencing return to
work. Br Med J 4:277, 1971

Roth JA, Eddy EM: Rehabilitation for the Unwanted. New
York, Atherton Press, 1967

RETARDED

Adams M: Social aspects of medical care for the mentally
retarded. New Eng J Med 286:635, 1972

Care of the mentally subnormal. Lancet 2:727, 1969
(Editorial)

Oppenheimer S: Early identification of mildly retarded
children. Amer J Orthopsychiat 35:845, 1966

SEX

Burt JJ, Brower LA: Education for Sexuality: Concepts and
Programs for Teaching. Philadelphia, W.B. Saunders Co.,
1970

Levin M: Healthy sexual behavior. Pediat Clin N Amer 16:
329, 1969

Masters W, Johnson V: Human Sexual Responses. Boston,
Little, Brown and Co., 1966

Rothchild E: Emotional aspects of sexual development.
Pediat Clin N Amer 16:415, 1969

Symposium on the physician and sex education. Edited by
SR Homel. Pediat Clin N Amer 16:322, 1969

SIGNS & SYMPTOMS

Signs and Symptoms: Applied Pathologic Physiology and
Clinical Interpretation. Edited by CM MacBryde, RS Blacklow.
Philadelphia, J.B. Lippincott Co., 1970

SOCIO-CULTURAL (also see ATTITUDES and VALUES)

Adair J, Deuschle K, McDermott W: Patterns and disease
among the Navahos. Ann Amer Acad Polit Soc Sci 311:86,
1957

Anderson JAD: A New Look at Social Medicine. London,
Pitman Medical Publishing Co. Ltd., 1965

Apple D: Sociological Studies of Health and Sickness: A
Source Book for the Health Professions. New York, McGraw-
Hill, 1960

Aring CD: Man versus woman: A historical and cultural
framework. Ann Intern Med 73:1025, 1970

Banfield EC: The Unheavenly City: The Nature and the
Future of Our Urban Crisis. Boston, Little, Brown and Co.,
1970

Baumslag N, Keen P, Petering HG: Carcinoma of the maxillary
antrum and its relationship to trace metal content of snuff.
Arch Environ Health 23:1, 1971

Benedict R: Patterns of Culture. New York, Houghton Mifflin
Co., 1934, p. 45

Boek WE, Boek JK: Health, social status and the life cycle.
J Chronic Dis 14:272, 1961

Brockington F: World Health. London, J & A Churchill,
1967, p. 47

Caudill HM: Night Comes to the Cumberlands. Boston,
Little, Brown and Co., 1963

Clark M: Health in the Mexican-American Culture. Berkeley,
University of California Press, 1959

Cultural factors in pediatric practice. J Pediat 78:547,
1971 (Editorial)

Cultural Patterns and Technical Change. Edited by M Mead.
Philadelphia, J.P. Lippincott Co., 1953

Culture and health disorders. Sociology in Medicine.
Edited by MW Susser, W Watson. London, Oxford University
Press, 1972

Deregowski JB: Pictorial perception and culture. Sci Amer
227:82, 1972

Dubos R: Man Adapting. New Haven, Yale University Press,
1965

Dubos R: The science of humanity. So Human an Animal.
New York, Charles Scribner's and Sons, 1968

Duff RS, Hollingshead AB: Sickness and Society. New York,
Harper and Row, 1968

Fry J: Medicine in Three Societies. New York, American
Elsevier, 1969

Gazaway R: The Longest Mile. New York, Doubleday & Co.,
1969

Gelfand: Medicine and Custom in Africa. London, E & S
Livingstone Ltd., 1964

Gist N, Halbert LA: Urban Society. New York, Crowell Co.,
1956

Haberman P: Ethnic differences in psychiatric symptoms
reported in community surveys. Public Health Rep 85:495,
1970

Handbook of Medical Sociology. Edited by HE Freeman, S
Levine, LG Reeder. Englewood Cliffs, Prentice-Hall Inc.,
1963

Henry J: Culture Against Man. New York, Random House, 1963

Hightower F: The goodliest land under the scope of heaven. American Surgeon 37:1, 1971

Jaco EG, et al: A month of illness and health care among low-income families. Public Health Rep 82:705, 1967

Jeffreys M: Social class and health promotion. Health Educ J 15:109, 1957

Kark SL, Stewart GW: A Practice of Social Medicine - A South African Team's Experience in Different African Communities. London, E & S Livingston Ltd., 1962

Kegeles SS: Attitudes and behavior of the public regarding cervical cytology: Current findings and new directions for research. J Chronic Dis 20:911, 1967

Knutson AL: The Individual, Society and Health Behavior. New York, Russell Sage Foundation, 1965

Koos E: The Health in Regionsville: What the People Thought and Did about It. New York, Columbia University Press, 1954

Lewis O: Children of Sanchez. New York, Random House, 1961

Martiney C, Martin HW: Folk disease among Mexican-Americans: Etiology, symptoms, treatment. JAMA 196:161, 1966

McDermott, et al: Introducing modern medicine in a Navaho community. Science 131:3395, 1960

McKeown T, Lowe C: An Introduction to Social Medicine. Philadelphia, F.A. Davis Co., 1966

Mechanic D: Medical Sociology - A Selective View. New York, Free Press, 1968

Michaelson M: Can a "root doctor" actually put a hex on or is it all a great put-on? Today's Health 50:38, 1972

Paul BD, Miller WB: Health, Culture and Community. New York, Russell Sage Foundation, 1955

The Planning of Change. Second edition. Edited by WG Bennis, KD Benne, R Chin. New York, Holt, Rinehart and Winston, 1969

Read M: Culture, Health and Disease. Philadelphia, J.P. Lippincott Co., 1966

Redlich FC, Hollingshead AB, Bellis E: Social class dif-
ferences in attitudes toward psychiatry. Sociological
Studies of Health and Sickness: A Source Book for the
Health Professions. Edited by D Apple. New York, McGraw-
Hill, 1960

Rogers CR: The characteristics of a helping relationship.
Personnel and Guidance J 37:6, 1958

Saunders L: Cultural Differences and Medical Care: The
Case of Spanish-Speaking People in the Southwest. New York,
Russell Sage Foundation, 1954

Sigerist on the Sociology of Medicine. Edited by MD Roemer.
New York, M.C. Publications Inc., 1960

Simmon LW, Wolffe HG: Social Science in Medicine. New
York, Russell Sage Foundation, 1954

Smith A: The Science of Social Medicine. London, Staples
Press, 1968

Some cultural aspects of transference and countertrans-
ference in individual and familial dynamics. Biological
Psychiatry Vol. I. Edited by JH Masserman. New York,
Grune and Stratton Inc., 1959

Stewart WH: A medical center culture. Roche Medical Image
9:No. 5, 1967

Watson W, Susser MW: Sociology in Medicine. Second edition.
London, Oxford University Press, 1971

Wight BW, Gloniger MF, Keeve JP: Cultural deprivation:
Operational definition in terms of language development.
Amer J Orthopsychiat 40:77, 1970

Wilner DM, et al: The Housing Environment and Family Life:
A Longitudinal Study of the Effects of Housing on Morbidity
and Mental Health. Baltimore, John Hopkins Press, 1962

STRESS

Society, stress and disease. Lancet 2:1125, 1971 (Editorial)

Stress and Disease. Edited by HG Wolff, H Goodell. Springfield, C.C. Thomas Publ., 1968

STROKE

Griffith VE: A Stroke in the Family. Harmondsworth,
Penguin Books, Ltd., 1970

SURGERY

Lewis C: Variations in the incidence of surgery. New Eng
J Med 281:880, 1969

TEAM (also see MANPOWER)

LiWang V, Bricker AJ: A team approach to teaching blind
homemakers: Home economist as a member of the health team.
Amer J Public Health 60:1910, 1970

Wise H: Primary care health team. Arch Intern Med 130:
438, 1972

TESTING

Lyman H: Test Scores and What They Mean. New York, Prentice-Hall, 1962

Oppenheimer S, Kessler JW: Mental testing of children under
three years. Pediatrics 36:933, 1963

THERAPEUTIC TRIALS

Lionel NDW, Herxheimer A: Assessing report of therapeutic
trials. Br Med J 3:637, 1970

TRANSPLANTS

Crosby DL, Waters WE: Survey of attitudes of hospital staff
to cadaveric kidney transplantation. Br Med J 4:346, 1972

URINARY INFECTION

Smellie JM: Acute urinary tract infection in children.
Br Med J 4:97, 1970

VALUES

Rogers CR: Toward a modern approach to values: The valuing
process in the mature person. J Abnorm Soc Psychol 68:160,
1964

VENEREAL DISEASE

Bender SJ: The venereal disease dilemma: A case in question. J Sch Health 41:105, 1971

Fiumara NJ: Venereal disease. Pediat Clin N Amer 16:333, 1969

Fiumara NJ, Lessell S: Manifestations of late congenital syphilis: An analysis of 271 patients. Arch Derm 102:78, 1970

Freeman CW: Case-finding in venereal disease control with special reference to the District of Columbia Dept. of Public Health. Med Ann DC 38:183, 1969

Schoelter AL: Gonorrhea: Diagnosis and treatment. Ann Intern Med 72:553, 1970

Wigfield AS: Attitudes to venereal disease in a permissive society. Br Med J 4:342, 1971

VISION

Binocular Visual Acuity of Adults: U.S. 1960-1962. U.S. National Center for Health Statistics. U.S. Public Health Service Publication #1000, Series 11, No. 3, 1964

Wilson RW: Characteristics of visually impaired persons, U.S. July, 1963 - June, 1964. Vital Health Statist 10:1, 1968

Index

false reactions   207-208

Ulcers, oral   278
Umbilical hernia   115
Urine culture   196
Uterine size   53-54

Vaccination   113
Vaginal
  bleeding   48
  carcinoma (estrogens)   39
  culture   195
  discharge   55
  smear   217-218
Vasectomy   72
Vernix caseosa   96
Vision testing   236
Vitamins   112

Water pollution   248
Weaning   111
Weight
  ideal   174
  infants and children   91
Well baby visits   89

Yucatan   18